HEART HEALTH FOR CANADIANS

Heart Health for Canadians

The Definitive Guide

Dr. Beth Abramson

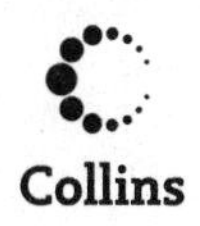

Collins

Published by Collins, a division of HarperCollins Publishers Ltd

First Edition

The information contained in this book may not be applicable in each individual case and should not be considered a substitute for the advice of the reader's personal physician.

This book draws on real cases from the author's 21 years of clinical practice. Some personal details have been changed.

HarperCollins books may be purchased for educational, business, or sales promotional use through our Special Markets Department.

HarperCollins Publishers Ltd
2 Bloor Street East, 20th Floor
Toronto, Ontario, Canada
M4W 1A8

www.harpercollins.ca

Library and Archives Canada Cataloguing in Publication
information is available upon request

ISBN 978-1-44340-502-7

Printed and bound in the United States

RRD 9 8 7 6 5 4 3 2 1

On a personal note . . .

To my mother, Dolores, a mentor and friend: I would not be where I am today without your tireless help.

To my father, Harry, a gentleman, scholar and role model: You have shown me what it means to be a real physician.

On a professional note . . .

To my patients and all those touched by heart disease: This book is for you.

CONTENTS

Part II: Preventing and Detecting Heart Disease

Part III: Navigating the System When Something Goes Wrong

HEART HEALTH FOR CANADIANS

FOREWORD

The best way to treat heart disease and stroke is to avoid them altogether, if possible. And it most certainly IS possible! But it's also hard to do. It's not just about eating the right foods, and the right amount of food, or getting enough exercise. The fact is, preventing cardiovascular disease is largely about what you can't feel or see. You can reach the danger point well before you notice any symptoms. In the absence of warning bells, many of us prefer not to change the habits that put us at risk. After all, you feel great, so what's the problem?

In *Heart Health for Canadians*, Dr. Abramson is determined to compel us to change, and to change now. In the following pages, you'll learn the specific, positive steps you can take to reduce your risk for heart disease and stroke as much as possible. And her advice couldn't be more timely:

- Heart disease and stroke take nearly one in three Canadians before their time.[1] This costs 250,000 years of life and nearly $21 billion to our economy every year.[2]

- Eighty percent of premature heart disease and stroke is completely preventable.[3]
- Many Canadians think heart disease and stroke afflict mainly aging white males. They think they're risk-free until they're older. The same misconception drives the assumption that advances in heart surgery mean they don't have to worry. On both counts they are dead wrong. Far too many Canadians succumb to heart disease because they underestimate its very real threat to their health—no matter what their age, gender or ethnicity.[4]

In these pages, Dr. Abramson tackles the disturbing facts of heart disease and stroke head-on. She is superbly qualified for this task, as a cardiologist at St. Michael's Hospital in Toronto and Director of its renowned Cardiac Prevention and Rehabilitation Centre. She has cared for thousands of patients over the past 20 years and is a valued spokesperson for the Heart and Stroke Foundation™. Her family has also been touched by death from heart disease, which makes her book even more compelling.

You'll see that this book places great emphasis on preventing heart attacks and stroke, and on reducing risk factors. The reason is clear. That 80% figure I quoted earlier is actually good news. With four out of five premature heart attacks and strokes being entirely preventable, the best way to deal with them is to live a heart-healthy lifestyle. This will greatly reduce the burden on our health care system and give Canadians more time with their friends and family. *Heart Health for Canadians* is a guidebook for all of us to become advocates for our own heart health. We can do this through healthier living, recognizing the symptoms of heart disease and managing our care by asking the right questions of our doctors and other health care providers.

You'll also learn what to do when a heart attack or stroke occurs. We know only too well from our research at the Heart and Stroke Foundation that it's all too common to delay treatment—with sadly devastating results. Dr. Abramson deals with this unfortunate reality, and her central recommendation bears repeating: Seek medical help quickly! As she says, do not think twice about going for care.

Being your own advocate is just as important once you enter the health care system. Often, our own fears and anxieties take over when we go for tests or enter a hospital. This makes it hard to make calm, rational decisions. The bottom line is that we need to advocate for ourselves and enlist family members or friends who will speak up on our behalf. To do that effectively, we need to know the questions to ask about tests, treatments, procedures and medications. Dr. Abramson's information and advice is invaluable in helping manage the stresses of dealing with the health care system.

Because Dr. Abramson is also the Director of Women's Cardiovascular Health at St. Michael's Hospital, she knows just how often women, in particular, will minimize the symptoms of a stroke or a heart attack, putting their jobs or tasks at home ahead of immediately calling either their doctor or 9-1-1. Many myths still exist about women not being as significantly affected by heart disease and stroke as men. The simple and shocking fact is that today more women than men die of heart disease and stroke. Women need to take care of their health and make it a priority. One way to do that is for them to learn the warning signs of a heart attack or stroke; in her chapter on women and heart disease, Dr. Abramson takes great care to explain this. As she says, "If we don't take the time to take care of ourselves, we won't be around to take care of others."

While health guides are not usually page-turners, Dr. Abramson has succeeded in making *Heart Health for Canadians* highly informative, accessible, enjoyable and, most of all, engaging. In a book filled with stories from her own family and her patients, she brings each point to life.

The Heart and Stroke Foundation is excited about Dr. Abramson's book. It fits in with our work over the last 60 years to raise awareness and turn the tide on heart disease and stroke. Our mission is "Healthy lives free of heart disease and stroke. Together we will make it happen." Dr. Abramson's work as a cardiologist, as a Heart and Stroke Foundation spokesperson and now as an author moves us one step closer to achieving that mission.

Of course, the real measure of worth of *Heart Health for Canadians* is the benefit you get from reading it. I hope you learn a great deal and gain the confidence to become a stronger heart-health advocate for yourself and your loved ones.

Here's to your heart health!

David Sculthorpe, CEO
Heart and Stroke Foundation

INTRODUCTION

For more than 20 years as a physician, I've believed in empowering patients and their families with information, advice and solutions. My job as a cardiologist is to help you understand the core issues that are relevant to your cardiac care. This is especially true if you're dealing with a new diagnosis or recovering from a health crisis, or if you simply want to take everyday steps to lead a healthier and more active life.

If you're holding this book in your hands, you are seeking just this kind of help.

That's why *Heart Health for Canadians* is a plain-language guide for everyone—a comprehensive look at the heart and its system of blood vessels and the many ways to take care of it all. Cardiac care may be cutting edge, but what you need to know can be broken down into simple concepts that anyone can follow. And since new research is emerging all the time, my mission is to help you discern the right questions to ask your health care professionals. The goal is to get on a path that makes the most sense for you.

Every one of you is different. Some have only a vague sense of what heart disease means. Others may have been told by a doctor that their blood pressure is too high, their cholesterol levels are abnormal, and they need to lose weight. You may know your grandmother died of a heart attack in her 70s, but you're not sure if that family history puts you at risk of developing the disease. (It doesn't, as we'll discuss in Chapter 2.) Or perhaps your experience with heart disease has been like a plunge into the deep end: You or someone you love was rushed to the hospital because of chest pains, setting off rounds of consultations, tests and procedures. In every case, you are thinking about your heart and contemplating the future with fresh eyes. With each day that passes, and each minute you spend waiting in a doctor's office, your list of concerns is piling up.

I wrote this book not just to answer common questions but also to put worried minds at ease. There are so many positive steps you and your loved ones can take right now to focus on heart health, no matter your age or the situations you're facing. I'll take you through the progression of heart disease and what you can expect at every stage and with every problem.

I've spent more than a decade as a spokesperson for the Heart and Stroke Foundation—and I've seen thousands of patients who decided to start focusing on their health after a point of crisis, such as a heart attack that left them with significant damage to the heart muscle. It's far less common to be proactive about heart health when you have no symptoms at all, but that's exactly when you or your family members can make a lasting impact. Studies show that up to 80% of heart disease is preventable. My mission is to help you make critical changes, as early as possible, to prioritize your heart health and take simple, proactive steps to establish a heart-healthy lifestyle. Prevention is about making small differences in our lives in order to foster long-term changes. In this hectic world, I realize it's very hard for all of us to work towards goals that seem intangible and down the road. But there *is* a payoff, and it's phenomenal.

If you have heart disease or are at risk of developing it, you need not only medicine but also motivation. Some readers may want to tackle long-standing goals—whether that's to stop smoking, to eat more healthily or even to visit their family doctor for an overdue checkup. I'll take you through the key principles and tools of prevention. We'll discuss everything that is in your power to change right now. You'll also learn what happens to the heart when something goes wrong, the tests doctors use and the treatments that correspond to each diagnosis. Ultimately, you'll see how vital a role you can play in shaping your future.

This book is comprehensive in scope, which means you don't need Google around for medical information about heart disease—a practice that can lead both to misinformation and information overload. But if you must search online, the two best sources of information are the Heart and Stroke Foundation (www.heartandstroke.ca) and the American Heart Association (www.myamericanheart.org). These sites will help you in your quest for credible information on heart health.

As a doctor and patient advocate, I want to drill down to the most essential information. Unfortunately, a great deal of misinformation exists about heart disease and stroke, in part fed by the many dubious blogs and websites out there full of mistaken beliefs and outdated statistics.

There are many common myths about who develops heart disease. For decades now, the average person has thought of heart disease in a narrowly defined way. In our minds, a "typical" victim of a heart attack or stroke is always a man past middle age—a stressed-out, sedentary person who eats a steady diet of burgers and fries. Most of us wouldn't include a woman in that profile, especially not a woman in the most active years of her life. Women develop breast cancer, the thinking goes. But they don't have heart attacks.

I've come across such misconceptions time and time again. As a clinician, teacher, and director of a cardiac rehab centre at St. Michael's Hospital in Toronto, I always reiterate one simple fact. Heart disease is an equal opportunity killer. It's a leading health threat to *all* Canadians, period. Men and women alike.

In fact, cardiovascular diseases—heart attack and stroke—are the number one killers internationally, accounting for 30% of all deaths. Around the world, this troubling trend affects both men and women at an equal rate, crosses all socio-economic levels and is perilously related to growing rates of obesity and smoking.

The latest statistics are astounding. According to the World Health Organization, of the 17.3 million people who died from cardiovascular disease globally in 2008, 7.3 million deaths were due to coronary heart disease and 6.2 million to stroke—which is the loss of brain function because of a lack of blood supply to the brain. And the numbers are only increasing: It's estimated that approximately 23.6 million people will die around the world annually by 2030 from cardiovascular disease. The tragedy is that many of these deaths are preventable if we attack the root causes, among them poverty and poor nutrition.

Even in a privileged country like Canada, we're not immune to the dangers. The Heart and Stroke Foundation estimates that there are 70,000 heart attacks and 50,000 strokes each year in this country—multiply that by 10 in the United States. In the time it might take for you to read a chapter of this book, one Canadian will have died from heart disease or stroke. In fact, cardiovascular disease accounts for one death out of every three in Canada.[1] The good news is that since 1952, according to the Heart and Stroke Foundation, deaths from cardiovascular disease have decreased by more than 75%. But on the other hand, a growing number of people are living with heart disease or surviving stroke. This causes a huge burden on our society. Heart disease and stroke costs the Canadian economy more than $20.9 billion each year in doctor services, hospital costs, lost wages, medications and decreased productivity.[2] Add to this the considerable personal toll, both emotional and physical, that the disease can take on you and your family members.

Every one of us, in one way or another, has a close connection to heart disease. I'm no exception.

I was born into a medical family, the daughter of a first-rate cardiologist. My father, Harry, taught me about the simple power of listening to his patients. I think everyone needs a doctor like Harry Abramson—thorough and uncomplaining, someone who understands that people need to be heard to feel they're cared for. My father didn't just treat heart disease; he experienced its effects in a deeply personal way. His own father, Ben Abramowitz, suffered for many years with angina, the chest discomfort that results when the heart is not receiving enough blood. When I was 14 years old, my grandfather Ben suffered a heart attack and died, leaving our family devastated. Over the years, my father and I often reflect on the fact that, were my grandfather to get sick today, the outcome would be very different. Today, a patient with severe angina might undergo a simple catheter procedure to unblock a damaged coronary blood vessel and then go home the next day. Treatments vary nowadays. Many people still imagine that heart procedures consist only of a surgeon cracking open the chest cavity. The new techniques can be minimally invasive and astoundingly precise; we'll cover them all in Chapters 10 through 12.

But before we get to treatments, it's imperative to know what exactly makes the heart function (see Chapter 1) and to recognize the warning signs that develop when the heart and its system of blood vessels are being compromised. Far too many people these days think if your heart is in trouble, you'll feel it in the most obvious way, as it's portrayed in the movies: You'll have an elephant on your chest. That's not always the case, which we'll explore in Chapter 5. In my practice, I see patients all the time who never imagined the symptoms they were experiencing—shortness of breath and a pain down the arm—were actually the warning signs of an impending heart attack.

The more aware we become of what heart disease looks and feels like, the more lives will be saved. In this book, no question is too silly and no term is left undefined. Although universal, all the medical concepts will be explored from a Canadian perspective. I want you to feel as if you have every base covered when you have that long-awaited appointment with your doctor. Our country has a fantastic health care system, allowing us to access the best experts around us. Patients and families need to be able to maximize their interactions with physicians—it's about feeling armed with the right information.

Think of this as the only crash course you'll ever need in heart disease and heart health. Hopefully, we can prevent this disease from reaching you or your loved ones. However, if it already has, we can equip you with a thorough checklist to take to your consultations. Protecting your heart health begins with you and the doctors you trust. Any well-informed support network is like an essential partnership. One person can't function without the others, and everyone has a stake in what lies ahead. Think of it this way: You're now part of a movement of heart-health advocates! And you thought you were just buying a book.

PART I

Understanding Heart Disease

1

ANATOMY OF THE HEART

"How does my heart work? Why do I need to know?"

The first step in learning about the heart is to look at what has to go *right* for it to function properly.

Let's begin with the word *cardiovascular,* which is actually quite easy to define once you break it down. In translating loosely from the Latin—may my high-school Latin teacher forgive me—*cardio* means heart and *vascular* means blood vessels. Therefore, cardiovascular diseases are those that involve the heart, the blood vessels and the system of blood flow. Understanding how the cardiovascular system works will help you better understand what's happening if something goes wrong.

Your heart is located in between your lungs in the centre of your chest. It's slightly to the left of your breastbone (sternum). I teach my residents that there are five main parts to the heart. Obviously it's more complicated than that, or I would be out of a job! But in the big picture, a patient is at risk when one of the following five parts of the heart breaks down or develops a problem: the muscle, the coronary arteries, the valves, the electrical system or the sac surrounding the heart.

Internal Anatomy of the Heart

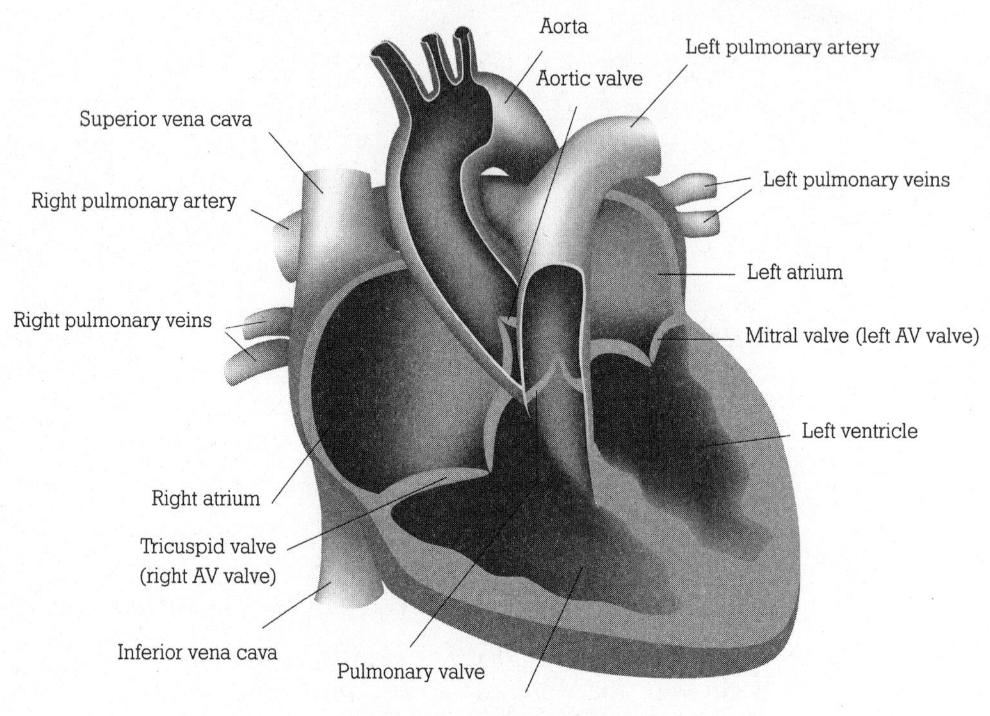

A real heart looks nothing like a drawing on a Valentine's card. It's actually the approximate shape and size of a fist. It weighs between 7 and 15 ounces and is divided into two pumping sides. The right side of the heart is where the "bad blood" (deoxygenated blood) enters from your body. You might remember this from science class. The left side of the heart is generally thought of as more important because it is the main pump that sends "good blood" (oxygenated blood) out to your body. Each side of the heart also has a top and a bottom. This means the heart is divided into four chambers: right atrium, right ventricle, left atrium and left ventricle. The bottom chambers—the ventricles—are the main pumping chambers. The top chambers of the heart—the atria—help coordinate and pump blood through to the ventricles. In between the chambers of the

Pathway of Blood Flow Through the Heart

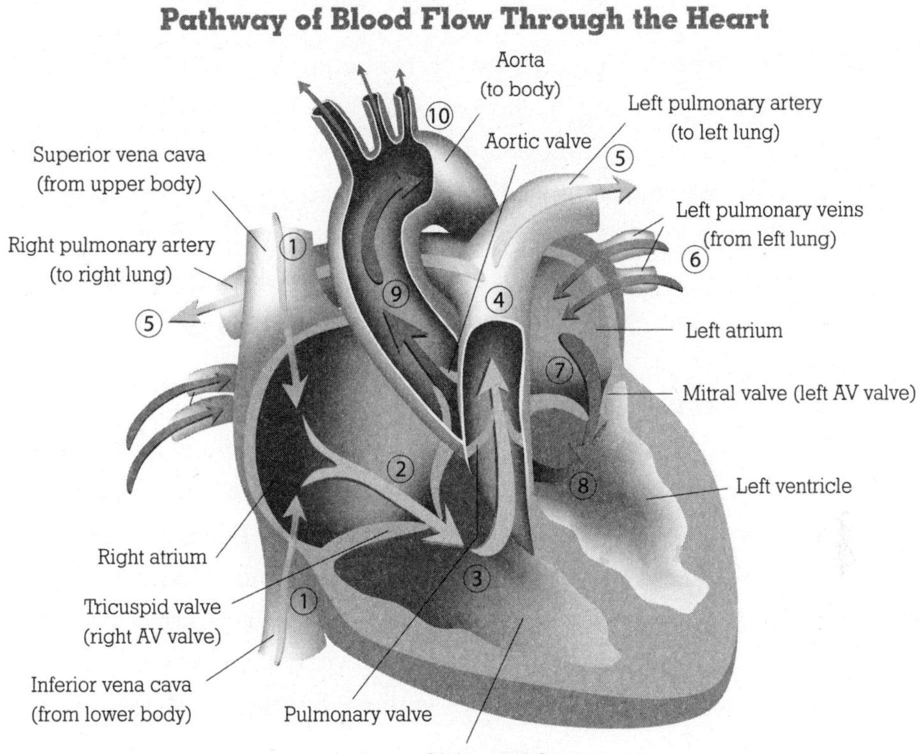

heart (as well as the entry from the heart to the lungs and to the aorta) are the valves.

The process of bad blood coming in and good blood flowing out works like this: The blood enters the lungs from the right side of the heart. To be more specific, the blood goes through the right atrium, across the tricuspid valve to the right ventricle, through the pulmonary valve, then on to the lungs. While in the lungs, the blood is oxygenated. The good oxygenated blood then drains back into the left side of the heart. The blood enters the left atrium, goes through the mitral valve, and enters the left ventricle. From the left ventricle, oxygenated blood is pumped to the rest of your body through the aortic valve, into the aorta.

I hope this isn't as confusing to you as it was when I first began studying medicine. I was 20 when I landed at the University of

Toronto's med school, after two years of undergrad. At the time, it would take me hours to read a journal packed with medical lingo that I read within minutes today. Of course, the more I studied, the more the core concepts became more accessible; and the more familiar the medical language became, the more the ideas came together. At any event, in this book we're just looking at the basics. Let's talk about each of the five parts in more detail.

The Muscle

The heart's essential role is to pump blood to the rest of the body, brain and vital organs. The main pumping part of the heart is muscle. It's called the myocardium. The other two main types of muscles in the body are the skeletal and smooth muscles. The heart muscle has special properties and cells that make it more resilient than the other muscle types, allowing the heart to beat for our entire lifetimes without becoming fatigued or burning out.

How do we describe the heart's efficiency? Medically, we use the term *ejection fraction.* Under normal circumstances, if you think of your heart as a cup, about half of the blood in that cup is ejected—or pumped forward—with every heartbeat. This amount is called the ejection fraction. If the heart muscle is weakened and the pump cannot work as efficiently, the ejection fraction is reduced. This is often seen in patients after large heart attacks and those with congestive heart failure (see Chapter 9).

❤ **You need to know: A normal ejection fraction, or EF, is in the range of 55% to 70%. A low EF is less than 55%. A very low EF (under 30%) is a serious problem.**

The heart muscle is not very thick—about 1 cm—and does not change in size under normal circumstances once you reach adulthood. However, several main things can go wrong with the muscle: It can die, weaken or become stiff and thicken. The most common cause of heart-muscle damage in the world is from a heart attack. If you have a heart attack, the blood supply to your heart muscle is cut off, and the heart muscle dies in the area of that decreased blood supply. A heart attack is the outcome of starving the heart of the essential oxygen and nutrients in the blood. It can cause weakening. A weakened heart can't pump blood efficiently. In contrast, heart muscles can also become abnormal—by thickening or stiffening rather than weakening—which can be caused by a variety of factors such as high blood pressure or diabetes. Both a thickening and weakening of the heart muscle can lead to congestive heart failure.

An average heart beats between 60 and 100 times per minute—on average, about 75. Multiply this by 60 and you get 4,500 heartbeats per hour, which is over 100,000 heartbeats per day. Continuing on with the math, multiplying by 365 days per year, that is almost 40 million heartbeats per year. Assuming a young life expectancy of 75 years of age, which is a gross underestimation, your heart is designed to beat more than 3 billion times in a lifetime. Each day, your heart beats and pumps thousands of litres of blood to the body.

You can help maintain a healthy heart muscle by keeping the arteries free of "junk"—a buildup of plaque, or atherosclerosis. Eat healthy foods, adopt a regular routine of activity, don't smoke, keep your blood pressure down and keep your bad cholesterol levels low.

The Coronary Arteries

A blood vessel—whether a capillary, vein or artery—carries blood through the organs and tissues of the body. Coronary arteries are the blood vessels vital to the function of the heart. They encircle the heart like a crown (hence the name, from the Latin *corona*). The coronary arteries branch off the aorta—the body's main artery—and supply the heart with blood to keep it alive. From the heart, the pulmonary artery takes the bad blood away to the lungs, where it is oxygenated. Then, other arteries pump the good blood into the rest of the body.

Arteries are complex organs. They have layers of cells, made up of muscle tissue and the endothelium, the important inner coating of arteries. The endothelial cells are like the EMS team of the arteries. They respond to distress by secreting substances to keep your blood vessels healthy and to protect you when those blood vessels are injured. For example, if you get cut, it's important that your body clots so the bleeding can stop. The endothelial cells release substances called factors that cause the platelets in the blood to gather and form a blood clot. Although it helps with a cut, a clot can be dangerous if you have disease within the blood vessels (such as atherosclerosis) or a buildup of cholesterol in the arteries. Clots in the arteries can interrupt the flow of blood. This is what occurs when you have a heart attack.

There are two main coronary artery systems that supply blood to your heart: the right and the left. The left main artery branches into two other arteries: the circumflex coronary artery and the left anterior descending (LAD) artery. A disruption of the left main artery is usually life threatening because it supplies most of the blood to your heart. The term used among physicians is that a disease of the left main artery is a "widow-maker lesion" or a "widower-maker," as the case may be.

The main coronary arteries all have side branches that also supply blood to your heart. If you have a heart attack, the location and extent of the heart attack is often determined by the artery that's blocked at the time. Damage will occur "downstream" from the blockage. That means if a block occurs in the artery, blood won't get past the block to reach the heart tissue downstream. This often affects the heart muscle that is supplied by the diseased artery and its side branches. So if the blockage is in the left main, then most of your heart would be affected. If in the right, usually the bottom part of your heart would be affected. This is why a left blockage is often more serious.

Arterial Supply to the Heart

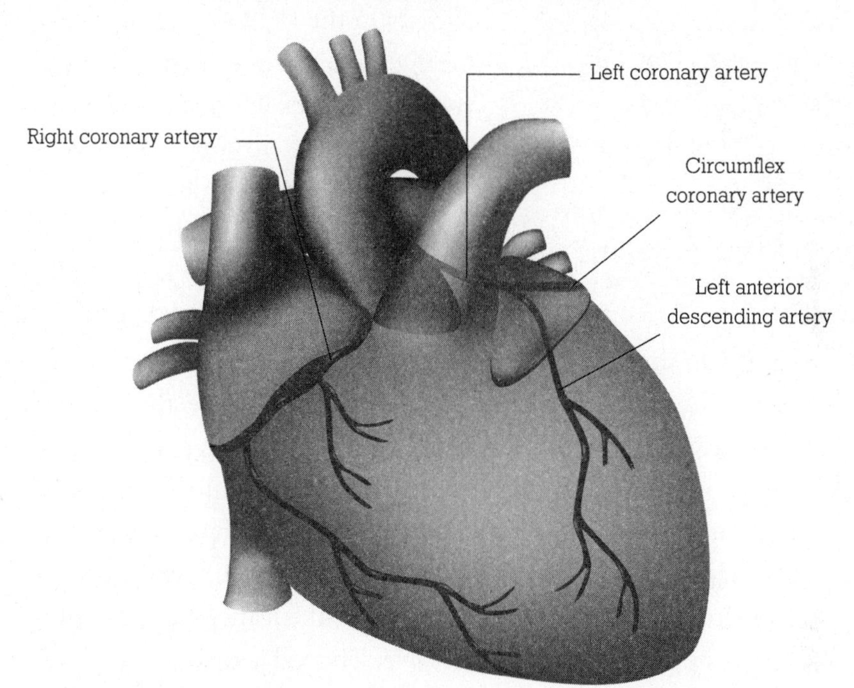

The main disease of the arteries is atherosclerosis, when junk builds up in your arteries. When this happens, the artery is at risk of becoming clogged because a blood clot can form in the vessel. With atherosclerosis, the blood flow to the heart is interrupted. This may lead to a heart attack, where the heart muscle downstream from this blockage is damaged. You might be treated for coronary heart disease with a procedure such as an angioplasty or bypass surgery (see Chapter 10). Don't worry. Soon, we'll discuss ways to prevent the disease from developing in the first place.

The most common cause of artery disease is atherosclerosis—the buildup of plaque. However, there are other unusual causes of artery disease that are beyond the scope of this book. For instance, you may experience artery disease because of inflammation of the arteries. This condition is rare and can be treated with anti-inflammation medications such as steroids rather than anti-atherosclerosis medications such as cholesterol-lowering drugs.

The Valves

The top part of your heart (the atria) is connected to the bottom part (ventricles) with valves. These are called AV valves, for "atrium" and "ventricle." On the right side of the heart, the AV valve's name is the tricuspid valve, and on the left side of the heart, between the left atrium and left ventricle, the AV valve is called the mitral valve. *Tricuspid* means the valve has three leaflets, or parts. A mitral valve is *bicuspid,* which means it has two.

Of all the heart's valves, your mitral valve is the most complex. This valve is made up of the papillary muscle, the chordae tendineae and the mitral valve annulus. All three parts need to work together to prevent problems with your mitral valve. The papillary muscles connect the valve to the left ventricle. The chordae tendineae are little pieces of the valve that attach to these muscles; they also join to part of the leaflets. The annulus is the top ring of the mitral valve. The valve opens and closes with blood flow going through the heart. If you were to look head on at a mitral valve, as we often do with an echocardiogram, it looks like a fish mouth opening and closing.

There are other main valves in the heart. The valve that connects the right side of your heart (right ventricle) to the pulmonary artery is called the pulmonary valve. The valve that connects the main left pumping chamber (left ventricle) to the aorta is called the aortic valve. The aorta supplies good, oxygenated blood to your entire body.

In the majority of people, an aortic valve has three parts, or leaflets. But up to 1 person in 200 is born with a two-leaflet, or bicuspid, aortic valve. In other words, they're missing a leaflet. It's a common congenital abnormality. ("Congenital heart disease," which is beyond the scope of this book, falls under the umbrella of pediatric medicine; it means the diseases of the heart we are born with.) Although a bicuspid valve can function very well, there is more wear and tear on it; over time, the valve can become worn and narrowed. Some people with bicuspid valves will need a valve replacement in their 50s (see Chapter 13).

When a valve is abnormal—that is, when it leaks or is narrowed—the blood flow through the valve is not as it should be. This turbulent blood flow can often be heard when a doctor examines a patient with a stethoscope. The sound heard from blood flowing through an abnormal valve is called a murmur. Sometimes, people are born with slightly abnormal valves that, over time, can wear out or require surgery. Not all murmurs are serious (see Chapter 9). Although valves can also become infected or wear down, these problems are generally less common than coronary artery disease.

Mitral valves can become narrow if they are inflamed by diseases such as rheumatic heart fever, or they can become leaky for a variety of reasons, including that the heart muscle is enlarged and stretching the mitral annulus (top ring). A certain number of people are born with a floppy mitral valve that looks thick and slightly abnormal. The valve can also back up, or prolapse, into the

When a valve leaks, the medical term is *regurgitation*. When a valve is narrowed, the term is *stenosis*. Not all leaky or narrowed valves are serious problems. In fact, with our modern technology, we can see natural leakiness, often reported as physiologic or mild regurgitation. If this term appears on an echocardiogram report (an ultrasound of the heart; see Chapter 7), it usually means nothing other than our instruments have been refined to pick up subtle variations on normal. When I am asked to see a patient for mild regurgitation on an echocardiogram, all the patient usually needs is reassurance.

left atrium. This floppy valve is often called a myxomatous valve. Over time, it can become more leaky. Not all myxomatous or prolapsing mitral valves, however, require treatment, but if a doctor discovers one, it needs to be monitored over time.

The Electrical System

You may be wondering what controls the pace of the heart as it pumps blood. In other words, what makes the heart beat? Most people don't know that the heart has an electrical system, somewhat like the wiring in a house. Specific cells in the electrical system of the heart carry electrical impulses, which result in the heart beating at an average normal rate of between 60 and 100 beats per minute.

In effect, the electrical impulses are causing your heart to contract in a coordinated fashion. When you think of a heart, the "lub dub" of every heartbeat is really due to the heart muscle contracting after the activation of the atrium and then the ventricle. It's actually the sounds of the various valves closing.

The electrical signals that set the contractions in motion begin at the top part of the right atrium in the sinoatrial (SA) node. This is sometimes called the heart's natural pacemaker. When the electrical impulses are released from the SA node, it causes the left and right atria to contract. The impulse then passes through to the atrioventricular (or AV) node, the spot in the heart where the electrical connections of the atria and ventricles meet. At the AV node, the signal is then sent along to the muscle fibres of the ventricles, causing them to contract.

The electrical nodes as well as some special electrical fibres of the heart have certain properties that keep your heart's electrical system in check. For example, at the AV node, there is a "stop sign." It's not actually a stop sign, but the tissue in the node possesses properties to prevent your heart from beating too fast.

A heart rate over 100 is a fast rate, or tachycardia (literally "fast heart"). A heart rate under 60 is a slow heart, or bradycardia. But remember that the normal rate of 60 to 100 refers to the average heart rate. It is entirely normal for your heart to race under times of stress, and you can even have spikes of high heart rates during the day. At night, it's normal for your heart rate to slow down when you sleep. Not to worry. It doesn't stop. Fitness can impact your heart rate. An athlete training for the Olympics will have a low resting heart rate, and if you are "medically deconditioned"—a polite way to say "out of shape"—your heart rate will be faster than someone who is athletically fit.

❤ **You need to know: It's normal for your heart rate to vary during the day. The more fit you are, the lower your resting pulse.**

Problems with the electrical system in the heart are called arrhythmias. Although there are exceptions to the rule, many arrhythmias are often not serious, which is why we call them benign in nature (see Chapter 9). Generally, electrical problems of your heart are less serious than problems with coronary arteries.

The Sac Surrounding the Heart

The sac surrounding the outside of your heart, otherwise known as the pericardium, is the least essential part of such a vital organ. You do not need the pericardium for normal heart-muscle function, and it may very well be something that has been left over as humans evolved. Some people are even born without one. Sometimes the pericardium can become inflamed or irritated. When this occurs, it's typically painful but not usually serious (see Chapter 9).

So we've worked our way from the inside of the heart to the outside, from the muscle, valves, arteries and electrical system to the pericardium. Now you have a sense of the heart's anatomy and how it has to function in order for you to thrive. Understanding these five parts of the heart is not intended to make you a doctor overnight, but it will help you see the all-important bigger picture.

2

PREDICTION AND RISK FACTORS FOR HEART DISEASE

"My grandfather had a heart attack at age 41. Am I at risk?"

The answer to that question is simple. Purely in terms of family history, you're not at risk. Risk applies when your most immediate relatives—a parent, sibling or child—have heart disease. Risk doesn't skip a generation, like from grandparent to grandchild. But that doesn't mean you're home free. Risk factors take many forms.

I often say that heart disease is due to bad luck, bad living and bad genes. You can't change your genes. But you can improve your luck by changing the way you live. I also say that most heart attacks aren't sudden—they take many years of preparation. The good news is that many of the leading risks of heart disease are preventable.

Other than family history, the major traditional risk factors for coronary disease are age, smoking, abnormal cholesterol levels, high blood pressure and diabetes.[1] Being overweight and inactive and having certain biological markers in your body, such as a biomarker for inflammation, can also put you at risk.

There's also the factor of stress. I've found that people tend to blame stress for a host of health issues, but to be honest, on its own, stress isn't a major risk for heart disease. This might be shocking to hear. Or maybe it's reassuring! The truth is, stress won't kill you. But how you deal with it might. If you are buried in tension because of your job or your family, and you pick up a pack of cigarettes or gain 25 pounds, this will increase your risk for heart disease. However, if you cope with the stress in a positive way—by going for a walk, cooking a healthy meal or escaping with a good book—then the risk evaporates. The one exception to the stress rule is in instances of major catastrophe. Studies show a traumatic event, like the loss of a family member, may be linked to risk of future heart attack. The bottom line is that, under normal circumstances, you can control your stress and therefore eliminate its impact on the more important risk factors of heart disease.

❤ **You need to know: Stress is *not* as strong a risk factor for developing heart disease as family history, smoking, abnormal cholesterol levels, high blood pressure and diabetes. It's not stress that will kill you, but how you deal with stress.**

Here, in no particular order, are the major risks and their defining characteristics.

Family History

Let's return to the question about the grandfather at the beginning of the chapter. The key thing to keep in mind is that if you have a first-degree relative—a parent, sibling or, heaven forbid, a child—with premature coronary disease, then the likelihood you will develop heart disease is increased. You're linked to the family members closest to you, and you can share with them high blood pressure, diabetes or abnormal cholesterol. In fact, if you have a close relative with early coronary heart disease—a mother or sister who developed the disease before age 65, or a father or brother who had it before 55—your risk is twice the general population's of developing future heart problems.

Countless times I've seen patients who worry about a strong family history for heart disease because their grandparents, aunts or uncles had problems with heart and stroke. If they don't mention their own parents on the list, it's good news. Be assured that your genes don't put you at additional risk unless you have a close relative with coronary heart disease.

Another fallacy is that the risk passed on in your family is sex-specific. That's not the case. It's not inherited solely by women from their moms or men from their dads. Studies show that anyone—man or woman—with a parent with heart disease has up to two times a greater risk of developing the disease than a peer with no family history.

I saw a woman in her 60s who was experiencing shortness of breath and chest pain. The chest pain was brought on when she was moving, walking or picking up heavy things. We call this exertional pain. It is brought on with activity and goes away with rest. This patient did not have a family doctor. In fact, her therapist referred her to me. She didn't smoke and didn't have diabetes, but it turns out that she did have a strong family history of coronary disease. Her father had his first heart attack at age 37 and heart bypass surgery in his 60s. She herself had experienced high blood pressure when she was pregnant with her first child. Now, years later, her kids had issues with high cholesterol. Although her symptoms were classic, she had been in denial that they could be related to her heart—when in fact so much about her family history pointed to her increased risk for heart disease.

The kind of heart disease your relatives had also affects your risk. The more concerning and common hereditary diseases are the plumbing-related problems of the heart. When we talk about coronary heart disease, that means things that can go substantially wrong with "plumbing" and blood flow. That includes atherosclerosis (junk in the arteries), angina (a feeling of chest pain and heaviness) and heart attack.

In contrast, a woman came into my office quite concerned about her health given that her son had had an episode of tachycardia, or a fast heart rate—often seen in otherwise healthy people. I explained to her that this is not coronary heart disease, and she was not at any greater genetic risk than the average perimenopausal woman. Having a family member who has a heart rhythm problem (arrhythmia), or who requires a pacemaker or heart valve surgery, is not related directly to coronary heart disease and does not put you at increased risk.

❤ **You need to know: If a close relative of yours had a heart attack, angina or other blood-flow problem of the heart, then you're at risk of developing the same. If you or a relative had a non-plumbing problem—like arrhythmia—you are not at increased risk for coronary heart disease.**

It gets trickier when it comes to pinning down whether or not your family history includes angina. *Angina* is the term we use for chest pain that develops from poor blood flow in the heart (see Chapter 8). In the past, patients (primarily women) were often mislabelled as having angina when they actually had chest pain for other reasons, such as acid reflux. When I take a patient's history and hear that his mother had angina or even a heart attack in her 30s or 40s but that she lived well into her 80s without any treatment, I question the diagnosis. It is not likely that a person with serious angina would live to be an octogenarian without being treated.

Age

Another non-modifiable risk factor is how old you are. Just as you can't change death or taxes, when it comes to heart disease risk, you can't change your age.

Your risk for heart disease and, for that matter, other chronic illnesses such as diabetes, cancer and stroke, increases as you get older.

I'm talking to you, Baby Boomers. The Heart and Stroke Foundation reports that approximately 1,000 Boomers a day will turn 60 in this decade, entering a prime age for heart disease and stroke. Approximately 1.3 million, or 21% of Canadians aged 45 to 59, have *already* been diagnosed with heart disease, stroke or high blood pressure (hypertension). As Boomers enter their 60s, the age at which heart disease rates markedly begin to climb, the proportion of people with heart disease will also increase. Forty-two percent of Canadians in their 60s report having heart disease, stroke or high blood pressure. More Boomers are set to be diagnosed, as population estimates show that the number of Canadians in their 60s will jump by 50% over the next 10 years, from 2.8 to 4.2 million.[2]

❤ **You need to know: Even though heart disease is not just a disease of aging, as Baby Boomers enter their 60s, they are a prime target for heart disease.**

Yes, the notions of "old age" are changing. We're living more active lives in our 70s and 80s. But nearly 33% of deaths due to cardiovascular disease occur *before* people turn 75, which is younger than the average life expectancy of 77.7 years. Roughly 7,700 Canadians who die from heart disease each year are under the age of 65.[3]

When it comes to age as a risk factor, it's important to note that there's a gender distinction: Women and men develop heart disease at slightly different stages in life. A man's risk of heart disease is higher at any age, but it's significantly more common for men to experience heart attacks from age 40 on. When it comes to the heart and blood vessels, a 40-year-old man is about as healthy as a 50-year-old woman on the inside.

As a rule of thumb, women are protected from coronary heart disease until after menopause, when the ratio of estrogen to testosterone changes. About 7 to 10 years after mid-life, women start catching up to men in terms of their coronary risk. So, since the average age of menopause is 51, a woman's risk starts to increase significantly in her 50s and 60s.

❤ **You need to know: Women generally start to develop heart disease after menopause (in their 50s) and men in their 40s. At the same time, younger women and men are still at risk. Heart disease is the number-one killer.**

Younger women: You're not off the hook! Heart disease and stroke are the leading health threats to *all* North American women, no matter the age. In fact, I see many women in their 30s or 40s in my practice. One of my long-standing female patients had a glamorous life in her teens and 20s, leading a career that required her to keep her weight in check. Later on, she endured a challenging marriage, which led her to gain a lot of weight. This was especially dangerous given the history of heart disease in her family. When she was in her 30s, she suffered a heart attack so massive that she was left with severe damage to the heart muscle. Today, she is doing better; she has lost weight and is active and plays baseball regularly. On the outside, she is a vibrant, energetic woman. But on the inside, because of the extent of damage to her heart, she has to constantly deal with the possibility of congestive heart failure. A simple cough, for her, can be a sign that fluid has collected in her lungs. It just goes to show that this disease can strike us at any age and regardless of gender.

Smoking

If you are under 40 and you've had a heart attack, it's likely that you smoke. If you continue to smoke after your heart attack, you are just making it easier to have another one. It's as simple as that.

Current cigarette smoking is a powerful independent predictor of having a cardiac arrest if you are living with coronary heart disease. According to the Centers for Disease Control and Prevention (CDC), cigarette smoking increases the risk of death for people with coronary heart disease by two- or threefold. On average, adults who smoke cigarettes will die 13 to 14 years earlier than non-smokers—260,000 men and 178,000 women in the United States each year.[4] The Heart and Stroke Foundation reports that more than 37,000 Canadians die each year as a result of tobacco use and second-hand smoke—that includes more than 10,000 from heart disease and stroke.[5]

❤ **You need to know: Cigarette smoking is a strong predictor of having a cardiac arrest if you have coronary heart disease.**

The amount of risk associated with smoking and having a heart attack or stroke is greatest when people start to smoke at a young age. Today, approximately 12% of all Canadians aged 15 to 19 years smoke cigarettes. This happens to be the lowest rate of smoking recorded for the age group since Health Canada began collecting the statistics for its Canadian Tobacco Use Monitoring Survey in 1999. But it still means there are 268,000 Canadian teens who identify as smokers—and that's a disturbingly high amount. Based on recent data, there are over 5,000 new cigarette smokers every day in the United States alone. Most are under 18 when they have their first cigarette. In fact, one in five smokers is likely to start smoking between ages 12 and 17. The U.S. Surgeon General reports that 80% of people who use tobacco began under the age of 18. Heart *unhealthy* habits, unfortunately, can start early.[6]

Globally, the World Health Organization estimates that tobacco kills nearly 6 million people each year; more than 5 million are users and former users, and more than 600,000 of those who die are non-smokers exposed to second-hand smoke.[7] Almost 1 billion men smoke worldwide compared with 250 million women.[8] There are marked regional differences. In South Africa, the Philippines, China, Iran and Portugal, the smoking rates are much lower in women than men. In contrast, in Canada, the United States, Australia and Iceland, the rate of smoking men is only slightly higher than that of women. The 2011 Canadian Tobacco Use Monitoring Survey showed that in Canada, 20% of men smoke and 15% of women smoke. The rates of smoking in Canada vary from coast to coast across the provinces, from a low rate of 14% in British Columbia to a high rate of 22% in New Brunswick, Quebec, Manitoba and Saskatchewan.[9] It's estimated that one-quarter of all coronary deaths in Canada are caused by smoking. Patients who survive heart attacks do have high motivation to quit, but relapse rates are also high.

So, how exactly is smoking bad for your heart?

To begin with, it lowers HDL, the good cholesterol that prevents the buildup of junk in the coronary arteries, a condition known as atherosclerosis. Tobacco smoke contains 4,000 chemicals, including nicotine, an addictive drug that boosts the blood's thickness (coagulability). When there's more coagulability, there's a higher risk for a blood clot to form in your coronary arteries. This can cause a heart attack. Nicotine also prompts a rise in the body's adrenalin, putting more pressure and demand on the heart to perform. It constricts the blood vessels so the heart is trying to pump blood into smaller tubes. It's like blowing up a tiny deflated balloon—it takes a lot of effort. In addition, adrenalin causes the platelets of the blood to become more sticky so that they form clumps (or aggregate), which can disrupt the flow of blood through the heart.

In young and middle-aged women, the risk of stroke may be related to the actual amount they smoke. Consider a study of more than 100,000 women aged 30 to 55, most of whom were health-conscious nurses. Those who smoked less than half a pack per day had a risk of stroke that was more than 2.5 times higher than the non-smokers. Heavier smokers who had at least 25 cigarettes per day had almost four times the increased risk of stroke.[10] Even non-smokers can have up to a 30% higher risk of heart disease if exposed to second-hand smoke at home or at work. Short exposure to second-hand smoke can cause the blood platelets to become stickier, damage the lining of the blood vessels and decrease flow to the coronary arteries, potentially increasing the risk of a heart attack. In the United States alone, over the last decade, 60% of children aged 3 to 11 were exposed to second-hand smoke.[11]

❤ You need to know: Exposure to second-hand smoke can increase your risk of heart disease by 30%.

Fortunately, as time marches on, smoking is becoming more taboo. My cardiologist father recalls making rounds in his hospital in the 1960s when he came to a patient in her 80s. She was

When it comes to making lifestyle changes, I'm a realist. While the cardiologist in me wants everyone to strive for perfect behaviour, I know that's not realistic. That's why I counsel my patients on moderation—a piece of cake now and then isn't the end of the world, as long as it's incorporated into a diet that is generally healthy. But there's one big exception—smoking. It gets zero tolerance. As far as I'm concerned, the only safe number of cigarettes to smoke is zero.

on oxygen and had difficulty breathing. When he walked into her room, she asked, "Doc, do you have a light?" as she pulled out a cigarette. As crazy as this may sound, hospitals actually had smoking areas many years ago. As recently as the 1990s, smoking continued to be in vogue, with smoking sections in restaurants commonplace. We've come a long way indeed. Today's smoking statistics show a glimmer of hope. In the 1960s, about half of Canadians over the age of 15 smoked cigarettes. Now the rate is 17%—a significant reduction due to public education, advertising bans and smoke-free legislation. Thankfully, it is no longer "cool" to smoke.

I don't consider myself a prejudiced individual, but I really get upset when I still see young people smoking, so much so that I have to tell them. Years ago, my "gift" for saying the first thing that comes to my mind almost created a family feud when I encountered some young smokers. I was out for a nice dinner on a patio with my family to celebrate my mother's birthday. There was no smoking within the restaurant, but it was allowed outside. A group sitting beside our table—mainly young women in their 20s—lit up in unison. I sat there seething and initially asked them to please smoke in the other direction. They were offended. The situation escalated, and I told them that I was a preventive cardiologist with an interest in women's health and that they were, in addition of offending my family, harming themselves and ruining their health.

Although heart health is universal—as are the ways to prevent heart disease, such as getting your cholesterol in check—the unit of measurement is not. If you are searching for credible information on cholesterol in the United States, the measurement is described in mg/dl. Americans often aim for LDL cholesterol less than 200 mg/dl (or an LDL less than 100 mg/dl if you have heart disease).[12] In contrast, in Canada and most other places in the world, such as Europe, the unit of measurement is mmol/L.

On reflection, I might have been a little too dramatic. But my medical perspective was spot on.

Cholesterol

I knew a patient who looked like a poster boy for health and athleticism. He was 52 and had a high-stress job, but he spent much of his free time in the outdoors. He was an avid cyclist. No one would have ever suspected he had dangerously high levels of cholesterol, a result of his other passion: an indulgent diet full of rich, fatty fried foods. Sometimes looks can be deceiving.

Stages of Atherosclerosis

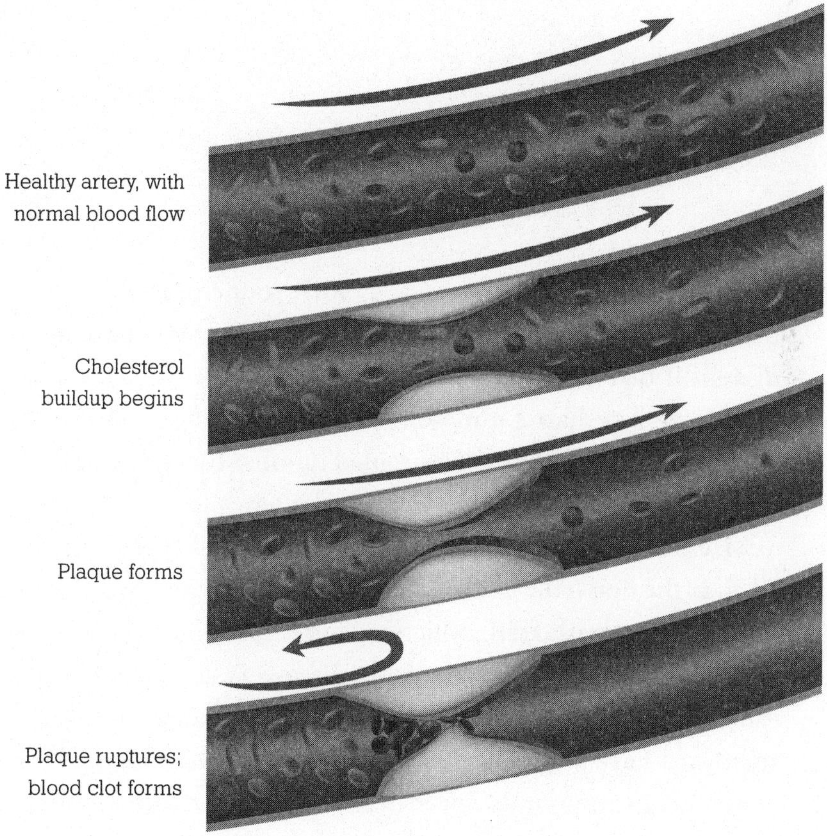

Healthy artery, with normal blood flow

Cholesterol buildup begins

Plaque forms

Plaque ruptures; blood clot forms

Cholesterol is a type of fat in your blood. It's used by your body to make cell membranes, vitamin D and hormones. There are two main types: low-density lipoprotein (LDL), or bad cholesterol, and high-density lipoprotein (HDL), or good cholesterol. LDL in high levels in the blood promotes the buildup of cholesterol (plaque) in your arteries. Plaque is not good. Think of plaque on your teeth. When this kind of plaque builds in the artery walls, atherosclerosis results—a dangerous narrowing of the arteries. HDL helps carry the bad LDL away from the artery walls and helps reduce plaque, making the arteries healthier. So having a low HDL puts you at risk for heart disease.

Like cholesterol, triglycerides are a type of fat found in the blood. High triglycerides are associated with obesity, alcohol consumption and increased risk of coronary heart disease. When people have high triglycerides, they often have diabetes or a low HDL level.

You might want to know exactly what your cholesterol "numbers" should be. It all depends on whether or not you have heart disease. If that is the case, in general, your doctor will want your LDL to be less than 2 mmol/L. Although the guidelines change from time to time, that's the accepted number for Canadians living with heart disease. Lower is always better.

Here's a handy trick to keep the cholesterol types straight: Look at the first letter in the acronym. LDL, which is bad, should be *low*. By contrast, HDL, which is good, should be *high*.

Cholesterol's impact on heart disease is considerable. It's estimated that if 10% of the population lowered its cholesterol, then we'd have a 30% decrease in coronary heart disease. That might mean thousands fewer deaths from heart disease every year.

♥ **You need to know: You should ask your doctor to check your cholesterol if you are a man over 40, if you are a woman over 50 or if you have other risk factors for heart disease.**

Checking your cholesterol is done with a simple blood test, usually while you are fasting first thing in the morning. You should ask your doctor to check your cholesterol if you are a man over 40; if you are a woman over 50 or postmenopausal; if you have had a stroke or have heart disease, diabetes or high blood pressure; or if your waist measures more than 102 cm (40 in.) for men or 88 cm (35 in.) for women. You also should have your cholesterol checked if you have a family history of premature coronary heart disease (see page 22).

Hypertension

Some time ago, I was writing a series of Ask Dr. Beth columns for the Heart and Stroke Foundation when the lawyer who reviewed the columns sent back a question: "What is hypertension?" Hypertension means high blood pressure. At the time, I was astounded that a person with multiple university degrees didn't know this. But I've learned that it's one of those medical terms that seem to be mystifying to many people.

Hypertension is known as a silent killer. That's because we can't feel our blood pressure—unless it is suddenly dangerously high or extremely low. I have had many patients tell me they know when their blood pressure is up, but to be honest, they really don't know. They are misinformed. You can't know what your blood pressure is without measuring it.

What exactly *is* blood pressure? It's an assessment of both the strength of the heart muscle pumping blood out of the heart and the healthiness of the arteries connected to the heart. Blood pressure—which varies from heartbeat to heartbeat—is the force exerted by the circulating blood upon the vessels, or the force on the walls of the arteries as blood circulates. You might be wondering if blood pressure is like the force of water coming out of a garden hose. In a way, it is. If the pressure is too high, the flowers you'll be watering will be destroyed. Ideal pressure allows the blood to flow freely through the vessels and deliver nutrients to the body.

In general, blood pressure is measured at a person's upper arm by a sphygmomanometer. The device consists of an inflatable cuff that briefly restricts blood flow and a device for measuring the pressure in the brachial artery (or artery in your arm). This artery is a branch of the major blood vessels, or aorta. On rare occasions, when someone is critically ill in the intensive care unit, we will measure blood pressure directly *inside* the arteries.

❤ **You need to know: Blood pressure can be elevated in one of two ways. The top pressure measured is called systolic pressure; the bottom pressure is called diastolic pressure. Systolic hypertension means the top number is too high; diastolic hypertension means the bottom number is too high. Some people have both numbers elevated.**

Blood pressure is described using two numbers. The top number (systolic blood pressure) measures the pressure when your heart beats. A normal value for the top number is less than 140. The bottom number (diastolic) is the measurement when your heart relaxes and refills with blood. The normal value for the bottom number is less than 90. What we consider "normal" can vary depending on whether blood pressure is measured at home or in your doctor's office. This is partly because you're more at ease at home and so your blood pressure should be lower, and you tend to be less relaxed when you visit your doctor.

A blood pressure (BP) of 120/80 represents a systolic pressure of 120 and a diastolic pressure of 80. The higher your BP numbers—either diastolic or systolic or both—and the longer those numbers are elevated, the more damage is caused to your blood vessels over time.

For most people, blood pressure should be less than 140 on the top (systolic) and less than 90 on the bottom (diastolic). But if you have an even lower blood pressure, achieved with lifestyle changes, then your risk for heart attack and stroke is decreased still. In a study of a large group of people followed for over 10 years, researchers found that high normal blood pressure (from 131/86 to 140/90) and normal blood pressure (from 120/80 to 130/85) still put people at increased risk for future heart attack and stroke compared with an optimal lower blood pressure (less than 120/80).

Blood pressure increases with age, for complex reasons. As you get older, the arteries can stiffen, or you may develop damage to your arteries from risk factors such as smoking and diabetes.

❤ **You need to know: In addition to causing stroke and heart attack, high blood pressure can lead to heart and kidney failure and is related to dementia, Alzheimer's and sexual problems. You can potentially prevent these issues if you control your high blood pressure.**

So how exactly can your blood pressure become a risk factor for coronary disease?

If your blood pressure is elevated over time, then you can see damage and disease in the arterial walls (atherosclerosis). The arteries can also become stiff. Both these problems can put you at risk of stroke—which is, essentially, a brain attack. Hypertension can lead to stroke because the pressures in your brain become too high, and you can bleed into your brain. This is called a hemorrhagic stroke. There are two types of stroke: Hemorrhagic stroke results from elevated blood pressure in the arteries. Ischemic stroke results from a lack of blood flow to the brain. A type of ischemic stroke called embolic stroke occurs when a piece of plaque that has built up in an artery flakes off (embolizes) and travels into the brain. High blood pressure in damaged arteries also leads to disease within the coronary arteries, which puts you at risk for heart attack.

Two Types of Stroke

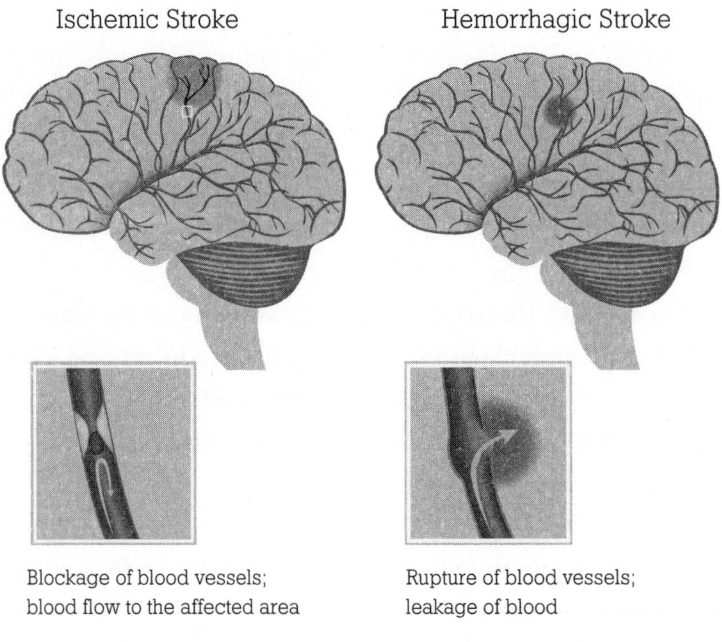

Ischemic Stroke

Blockage of blood vessels; blood flow to the affected area

Hemorrhagic Stroke

Rupture of blood vessels; leakage of blood

In medical terms, we call the risk of high blood pressure continuous, or linear—that is, the higher your blood pressure, the higher your risk of dying from heart disease and stroke. High blood pressure tends to run in families, so if you have a parent or sibling with high blood pressure, you are at increased risk of developing hypertension and need to get your blood pressure checked more frequently.

Hypertension is a major public health burden—it's estimated to cause more than 7 million (or roughly 13%) of all deaths worldwide.[13] A staggering 4.6 million Canadians between the ages of 20 and 79 have high blood pressure.[14] That is one in five Canadians! By the time we reach age 55, we have a 90% chance of developing high blood pressure. Hypertension is of particular concern to women, given the association with stroke. Each year, approximately 40% more women than men die from stroke in Canada—a trend we see internationally. It's important to note that as a woman ages and goes through mid-life and menopause, her risk of high blood pressure also increases.

I'm amazed by the number of times I'm asked to see a patient with new-onset or difficult-to-control hypertension, and that person doesn't know his family history. You may not want to talk to your parents or siblings about certain topics—but hypertension should not be one of them. Ask your parents and siblings if they are on blood pressure medications—it might make the difference for you in preventing high blood pressure yourself!

❤ **You need to know: High blood pressure is the leading risk of death in women and the second leading risk of death in men. It affects one in five Canadians.**

Lowering blood pressure through lifestyle, diet and, where necessary, medication is very important in reducing your chances of heart attack and stroke (see Chapter 4).[15] If you decrease your blood pressure by a mere 10 systolic points or 5 diastolic points, you can reduce your risk of developing a heart attack by 15% and risk of dying by 10%. According to Hypertension Canada, reducing your blood pressure by a relatively small amount can reduce your risk of heart failure by 50% and stroke by up to 40%.

Medications are usually needed for a systolic blood pressure of

160 or more or a diastolic pressure of 90 or more. However, what is acceptable as a normal blood pressure for an otherwise healthy person may not be what doctors accept as "normal" if you have heart disease, diabetes or kidney disease or have had a stroke. In these cases, doctors know to be more aggressive with blood pressure targets. If you are living with diabetes or kidney disease, we often recommend blood pressure to be less than 130/80. This is because higher blood pressure is even more dangerous if you have other health issues.

❤ **You need to know: You need medications for a blood pressure of 160/90 or higher. For most people, blood pressure should be less than 140/90.**

I have always advocated, as has the Heart and Stroke Foundation, for people to know their numbers. It's not good enough to go to your family doctor for an annual exam and be told your blood pressure is "okay." Ask your doctor what the numbers are, if they fall in a healthy range and what can be done to make them healthier. Everyone needs to have their blood pressure measured regularly at least once a year. Even local drug-store machines tend to be accurate. But remember: Having a few high blood pressure readings does not necessarily mean you have hypertension. A doctor will be able to diagnose you, usually after the course of several visits and readings. Be proactive, check your blood pressure regularly, know the actual numbers and ask your doctor what to do to make them even lower.

Sometimes people become nervous when they see the doctor. The term *white coat hypertension* refers to elevated blood pressure readings—triggered by the anxiety of a doctor's visit—in those who, on average, are in the normal range. This can be diagnosed easily, and true high blood pressure ruled out, with modern 24-hour blood pressure monitors.

A final bit of bad news here: If you have high blood pressure, you are more likely to have other risk factors for heart disease. Hypertension is the tip of the iceberg with heart disease risk. More than 90% of people living when it comes to high blood pressure have at least one additional risk factor for heart disease such as high cholesterol, diabetes or smoking. The good news is, these risks can be modified.

Diabetes

Diabetes is the disease that occurs when the blood's glucose (or sugar) levels are too high. If you have high blood sugar, you are at risk of developing coronary heart disease. High blood glucose levels can contribute to an increase of plaque (atherosclerosis). In other words, diabetes lays the groundwork for a heart attack.

Diabetes can develop in pregnant women, but the main types of the disease are juvenile diabetes (type 1) and adult-onset diabetes (type 2). Children and teenagers develop type 1 diabetes when the pancreas has problems secreting insulin, the hormone in the body that lowers blood sugar and keeps it under control. People with type 1 diabetes are usually not overweight. They need insulin injections to survive, but generally they have a lower risk for heart disease than people with type 2 diabetes, at least in the short term.

Adult-onset diabetes, which is linked to obesity, is eminently preventable. But it's become an epidemic in North America, a continent awash in mass quantities of high-calorie and unhealthy food. People with type 2 diabetes are unable to process or handle the insulin the pancreas makes. They're commonly heavier and inactive. They'll often needs pills (but not always insulin injections) in addition to diet and lifestyle changes to control their blood sugar. Diabetes pills can increase insulin sensitivity—meaning they make the insulin in your body work better. Others prompt the pancreas to produce more insulin.

❤ **You need to know: Adults with diabetes caused by unhealthy lifestyles are two to four times more likely to have heart disease or a stroke than adults who do not have diabetes.**[16]

Now here's the scary part. Although we call type 2 diabetes "adult onset," with increasing obesity rates, doctors are seeing children and teenagers with this type of diabetes. It's a trend we seldom encountered 20 years ago.

The diabetes risk is considerable. A patient with diabetes is at *the same* high risk for future heart attacks as someone who already has heart disease. Doctors call this being "risk equivalent." And if you have both heart disease and diabetes, the likelihood of a future heart event is significantly higher than it is for the average person with heart disease.

Although it has an impact on both sexes, diabetes is an even greater concern for women. Compared with a woman without diabetes, a woman with type 2 diabetes has an eight times increased risk of heart disease. In fact, diabetes takes away the protection that younger, premenopausal women have from developing heart disease at a young age.

The bright side is that change is entirely possible. Heart-healthy behaviour, regular activity and maintaining a healthy body weight can reduce the risk of diabetes.[17] I've seen many patients whose need for pills or insulin either is minimized or goes away with weight loss and exercise.

If you are at higher risk and have diabetes, it's very important to check your blood sugar and blood pressure regularly. I'm a fan of the home blood sugar monitors. Most of all, I believe in the power of lifestyle change, chiefly healthy eating and activity, to help control your risk factors. I can't stress these enough!

Weight

When you are overweight, your body does not process fat or sugars well, which can lead to damage or the buildup of junk in your arteries. Overweight people not only have a risk of blood-flow problems in the heart but also are susceptible to developing high blood pressure.

If you are obese, your life expectancy will be lower. If you weigh a third more than your optimal weight—which, for most North Americans, means carrying 50 to 60 extra pounds—you may shorten your lifespan by three years.[18] This may be partly because if you are overweight, you tend to be a couch potato and lead a sedentary lifestyle.

Not everyone who is carrying extra weight, however, is at increased risk of heart disease. It's important to consider the highly unrealistic body images foisted on young women and girls. The anorexic fashion model who is smoking and not exercising but looks "good" is actually dangerously unhealthy on the inside. In contrast, a young girl who is 5 to 10 pounds overweight but does not smoke, eats a balanced diet with fresh fruits and vegetables and is active is not at increased risk. She is "healthy on the inside" when it comes to her blood vessels. That being said, being 20% or more over your healthy weight is associated with a sedentary lifestyle and a diet high in fat.

We assess whether people are overweight in two main ways: through the calculation of body mass index (BMI) and by measuring waist circumference. BMI is calculated by dividing weight (in kilograms) by the square of height (in metres): weight ÷ (height x height) = BMI.

For instance, if you weigh 60 kilograms, or 132 pounds, and you're 1.6 metres tall, or 5 foot 4, then your BMI is 23.4. (Remember to figure out the squared height first, and then divide the weight by that number. In this case, multiply 1.6 by 1.6 [height^2], which equals 2.56. Then divide 60 [weight] by 2.56, which equals 23.4, your BMI.) If you weigh 200 pounds and are 6 feet tall, then your BMI is 27.1. BMI in the range of 25 to 29.9 is considered overweight. A BMI of equal to or greater than 30 is considered obese.

Rather than do the math yourself, you can use a simple online tool provided by the National Heart Lung and Blood Institute, a leading U.S.-based organization. The tool is at www.nhlbisupport.com/bmi. Just enter your height and weight, and it will calculate your BMI for you.

> You don't have to be a skinny mini to be healthy on the inside. Although obesity is associated with risk for heart disease, you can be a few pounds overweight and still be healthy on the inside if you are physically active, don't smoke and eat lower-fat, heart-healthy food.

For some muscular people, BMI might not be an accurate reflection of being overweight. That's where the waist circumference comes in. According to the Heart and Stroke Foundation, if you are Caucasian, Mediterranean or Middle Eastern, you should be concerned if your waist measures 102 cm (40 in.) or more in men, or 88 cm (35 in.) or more in women. At those measurements, you are at increased risk of developing diabetes, high blood pressure, heart disease and stroke. If you are Asian or South Asian, then the waist measurement danger level is 90 cm (35 in.) for men and 80 cm (32 in.) in women.

When doctors look at your body shape, they'll consider your waist–hip ratio. As women's magazines tell you, if your waist is larger than your hips, you are apple-shaped, and if your hips are bigger than your waist, you are pear-shaped. Women tend to gain weight around their hips in a pear-like distribution, whereas men tend to gain weight around their bellies. The good news is that extra weight on the hips does not put you at risk for the development of heart disease, diabetes, high blood pressure and high cholesterol. That's because the body processes fat differently around the belly. Belly fat can be composed of dangerous "inner fat." That is, a specific type of fat that goes in between your organs in your midsection. The bad news is that you can be a pear but you can't be a *big* pear—if you have a big waist and bigger hips, that doesn't protect you.

As a woman goes through midlife and menopause, fat distribution tends to change. Women can go from pear-shaped to apple-shaped with weight gain—but this is preventable. Getting rid of a "spare tire" or beer belly is important. The guidelines say that Caucasian women should have a waist circumference less than 88 cm (35 in.). Men's waists should be smaller than 102 cm (40 in.). Asian or South Asian individuals may need to have a smaller waist circumference to protect against heart disease and stroke. If your waist circumference is larger, it's important to know your other risk factors, such as blood pressure, cholesterol and blood sugar. And it's vital to lose weight.

How much you weigh can make a difference from an early age. A recent study[19] looked at 600 children and young adults from ages 6 to 20 and from a variety of ethnic backgrounds. The results showed that the heavier the child, the more likely she was to have carotid intimal-medial thickness, the measurement of the thickness of the artery, a marker for future heart disease. From my perspective, this research underscores the need for ongoing promotion of heart-healthy behaviour. It's never too late to make a lifestyle change. It's never too early, either.

Being overweight has a staggering impact on heart health. If you're overweight, you are more likely to have high cholesterol in the blood, especially high triglycerides and LDL cholesterol. You have a greater tendency to develop high blood pressure and type 2 diabetes. You are more likely to have metabolic syndrome, a grouping of weight-related major risk factors for heart disease including abnormal cholesterol levels (low HDL, the good cholesterol), high blood pressure and pre-diabetes (insulin resistance). People with metabolic syndrome have a higher risk of heart disease and stroke than people who have high blood pressure or high cholesterol who are not overweight.

Nearly one-quarter of Canadian adults, or 5.5 million people, are obese, and an additional 35% (8.6 million) are overweight. It's worse in the United States, where 144 million adults are overweight and one-third of U.S. adults are what we describe as medically obese. Men and women of all races and ethnic groups in the population are affected by this epidemic. Nearly one-third of Canadian children and adolescents are either overweight or obese according to Canadian Health Measures Survey data. Recently, I saw a 19-year-old in my office in order to assess his hypertension. It turns out that his high blood pressure had a direct relationship to his heavy weight. At 5 feet 8 inches tall, he weighed more than 200 pounds, putting him at risk for heart disease. His case speaks to the reach of the obesity epidemic. When I started my practice 20 years ago, I did not see teenagers with weight-related health problems. Now I do.

❤ **You need to know: If you are overweight, you are at risk of having metabolic syndrome, a grouping of major risk factors for heart disease including abnormal cholesterol, high blood pressure and pre-diabetes. People with metabolic syndrome have a higher risk of heart disease and stroke.**

Sedentary Lifestyle

Of all the risk factors for heart disease and stroke, physical inactivity is the most commonly seen in the population. Sitting on the couch for hours is detrimental to your heart health. If you don't engage in regular activity, you will be more prone to obesity, high blood pressure, and high cholesterol in the blood (triglycerides and LDL, or bad cholesterol), and you're even at risk for diabetes (high blood sugar levels).

The human body is better off being active, not sedentary. We need regular movement to keep the heart healthy and the cardiovascular system pumping effectively, especially if we are living in a world of unhealthy food choices. That said, not all sedentary behaviour has the same impact on activity levels. Watching television may be more dangerous for heart health than reading, for example.[20] Studies also show that as the hours of watching television increase, the more likely people are to engage in unhealthy behaviour such as snacking and overeating, and the more likely they are to be overweight.Readers tend not to snack as much!

According to the Heart and Stroke Foundation, almost half of Canadians are not as active as they should be. An overwhelming 91% of children and youth are not meeting physical activity guidelines. Children report spending twice as much time in front of a screen as they do engaged in physical activity. It's estimated that if Canadians were to increase their physical activity by 10% over a five-year period, we would save the Canadian health care system $5 *billion* in lifetime costs. So if you're walking 20 minutes a day, adding an extra 2 minutes a day and keeping it up could make a difference.

Inflammation and CRP

Think about a cut on your finger or falling down and bumping your knee. Whenever a part of your body is injured, it can turn red and swell. That's due to inflammation, when the body releases chemicals and white blood cells to the affected area in order to help it heal. But while inflammation can be good for the body, researchers believe it may also lead to the development of heart disease. Why? Because the inflammation can damage the walls of the blood vessels.

To find out if you may be at risk, you can take a simple

blood test to measure your CRP, or C-reactive protein, a marker for inflammation—although the test is not recommended for everyone. If you already have heart disease, or you're at low risk for developing the disease, the test will not usually provide your doctor with any more information than you already know. The important thing to remember is that inflammation in the body has many causes. I was at a medical convention a while ago and had my CRP level measured. That's what doctors do for fun at conventions: go for tests! To my surprise, the CRP measure was quite high. I was a little worried and took it up with one of the leading experts in CRP, a physician I know from Boston. In the end, however, I didn't have to be concerned about my heart. It turns out I had an untreated back injury that was the true cause of the inflammation. If you stub your toe, tear a ligament in your knee skiing, as I also did several years ago, or have a common cold, your CRP will be high. A high CRP in this context does not mean you are at increased risk for heart disease. Various other conditions raise CRP such as high blood pressure, obesity, smoking, having metabolic syndrome or being on hormone replacement therapy. The flip side is a recent study that identified women over the age of 60 and men over age of 50 with an elevated CRP but average cholesterol levels; when these people were put on cholesterol-lowering medications, their risk of heart attack, stroke, angina and death decreased.[21] Lowering your blood pressure, losing weight, exercising, stopping smoking and, when you can, stopping hormone replacement therapy also lowers CRP. You don't need a blood test to tell you that.

The bottom line for testing is this: We shouldn't measure CRP in everybody. Since risk factors increase with age, measuring a 40-year-old's CRP isn't always revealing of the future risk of heart disease. Younger people with no other risk for heart disease may not gain any insight from CRP. They are still at low immediate risk, even if the CRP is elevated. In addition, if you are already living with heart disease, or have had a previous stroke or blood vessel disease (circulation problems, peripheral arterial disease), you do *not* need your CRP measured. We already know you are at high risk. Knowing the CRP in this case doesn't change the fact that you are at risk and will need specific treatment such as cholesterol medication.

A young woman walked into my office because her family doctor was worried that her CRP was high and that she might be at risk for heart disease. I took her history and found out that she had had cancer. Before I could even think about her heart disease risk, I asked her to talk to her doctors to make sure there was nothing else serious going on. It turned out that her inflammation was not heart related.

Measuring Your Risk

Fortunately, no one single risk factor is responsible for developing coronary heart disease. In fact, usually multiple factors put you at the greatest risk over time. Doctors will look at a combination of every risk to calculate your future risk for heart disease. The process involves using a global risk assessment scoring system. In other words, doctors add up various risk factors, with slightly different weightings for each factor, and come up with a general prediction of their patients' heart disease risk.

North America's most common global risk assessment scoring system is the Framingham Risk Score, which was developed after a long-term study of individuals in Framingham, Massachusetts.[22] There are limits to this scoring system, since the Framingham population was white and working class. Nowadays, we will often adjust the score to take into account one's ethnicity. There is also a concern that the Framingham score underestimates risk in women. All the same, a Framingham risk scoring system is a good place to start.[23]

The Framingham Risk Score calculates your risk of heart

disease by considering your gender, age, cholesterol levels, smoking status, diabetes status, blood pressure and family history of the disease. If you have excess weight across the belly—the spare tire—then your risk is even greater. After compiling the pertinent information about you, your doctor can calculate how likely it is that you will develop heart disease and stroke over the next 10 years. Low risk is considered a less than 10% risk of developing heart attack or stroke in the next decade. Your doctor will worry if your risk is moderate (10% to 20% over 10 years) and certainly if it's high (more than 20% over 10 years). If you have an immediate family history of heart disease (see page 22), this risk is generally doubled—so if your Framingham score is 14%, your risk for developing heart disease will become 28%. Family history alone can move the risk from moderate to high. The good news/bad news is that young age tends to protect you significantly from developing coronary heart disease; being in mid-life and older puts you at an increased risk. If you use a Framingham risk scoring system and you are a premenopausal woman, by and large your risk will not be very high.

It's vital to ask your family doctor to review your risk factors for heart disease at your annual health exam. Women need to understand that a yearly exam should include much more than a mammogram and a pap smear. You should have your cholesterol checked, talk about your blood pressure, discuss any weight issues and review your family history. If you are young, or if you are a premenopausal woman with no risk factors for heart disease, there is no need to have your Framingham Risk Score measured at every annual checkup. If your doctor determines you are at low risk of future coronary disease, then it's recommended that you have your Framingham Risk Score calculated every three years. However, if you have an immediate family member with early heart disease or have one or more risk factors for heart disease, your doctor should check your Framingham Risk Score annually.

You may have noticed I haven't suggested any high-tech intervention for screening for heart disease, such as a total body CT scan or a calcium score. These are expensive and unproven methods for assessing your future risk. Besides, visualizing atherosclerosis (junk in the arteries) doesn't tell us exactly what your risk is for future heart attack. It just tells us your risk is higher than average. The corollary is that seeing "clean arteries" with an angiogram is not a get-out-of-jail-free card—there can be disease that is not visible to the naked eye.

The bottom line is that risk prediction is just that: *prediction.* Your doctor may identify a series of concerning risks, whether you have hypertension, a family history of early coronary disease or too much weight around the midsection. You already know that smoking is bad for you at any stage of life and that spending hours in front of the television with bowls of potato chips is not great for your heart. You know the benefits of adopting a lifelong approach to healthy behaviours. The question is, what steps can you take to make your heart health a reality? (That's what we'll discuss in Chapter 4.) The best you and your physicians can do after identifying your risk factors is to use the information to plan a course for the future, and you need to do this as a team.

What are the most common roadblocks you may encounter on your path to heart health? Do you make time for heart-healthy exercise every day? Do you see your family

Doctors can tell you if you have plaque in your arteries by performing a coronary angiogram (see Chapter 6) and subsequently a special ultrasound for the arteries called an intravascular ultrasound (IVUS). However, this approach is invasive and neither safe nor realistic to perform as a routine screen on everyone. More importantly, visualizing atherosclerosis doesn't tell us exactly what your risk is for a future heart attack. It just tells us your risk is higher than average.

doctor for regular checkups? Are you in a healthy weight range? Do you have enough balance between work and downtime? To succeed at addressing your risk factors for heart disease, you have to answer "yes" to most of these. It's challenging for everyone. But there's one group for whom this is a consistently difficult area: Of course, I'm talking about women. One of the most troubling facts in medicine is that more women are dying of coronary heart disease than ever before. In fact, women and men are now dying of the disease at an equal rate. What concerns me further as a cardiologist is that our awareness of the issues related to heart disease in women is an uphill battle. There are widespread (and false) beliefs that women are not as prone to heart disease as men, or that they have different symptoms of the disease than men. To help reduce the likelihood that women will be marginalized in their cardiac care, we have to correct these false impressions. We must also examine the issues related to women and heart disease.

3

WOMEN AND HEART DISEASE

"What are the heart disease risks for women, and how do they differ from those for men?"

This is a question I get asked constantly, as I often speak to patients and fellow physicians about issues related to heart disease in women. I find I spend much of my time on this subject dispelling misconceptions. Frankly, I've heard all kinds of gender-specific theories about heart disease. In the extreme case, there are patients who believe that *only* men have heart attacks. Most wouldn't go that far, but they'll tell you that when women do have heart attacks, they have entirely different symptoms than men. I can assure you: This is generally not the case (as you'll read when we cover symptoms in Chapter 5).

If I can share one main teaching point it's this: Women are more similar to than different from men—at least when it comes to their hearts. I can't stress enough that we have to start thinking of heart disease as both a male and female problem. In reality, heart disease and stroke account for nearly one-third of the deaths of Canadian women. In terms of the effects of the disease, women are much more similar to men than we acknowledge. The only major gender difference is that men tend to develop heart disease earlier in life than women do. Women are generally protected from the disease until they reach menopause, when estrogen levels begin to decline in the female body. Researchers have many theories why estrogen is a defence against heart disease. The hypothesis is that estrogen, which young women have plenty of, protects their arteries from being damaged. This is believed, in part, to be linked to estrogen's influence on regulating cholesterol levels in the body. Estrogen—the sex hormone produced in the ovaries—has a relaxing (dilating) effect on the arteries as well. Estrogen also decreases LDL (bad) cholesterol and increases HDL (good) cholesterol. With a change in her estrogen after menopause, particularly in her 50s and 60s, a woman's risk begins to rise as her risk factors for heart disease tend to increase. After menopause, body fat distribution changes, and women have a tendency for high blood pressure (hypertension), diabetes and increased cholesterol levels.

This may seem like a "free pass" for younger women, but it shouldn't be perceived as such. Even if you are in your 20s and 30s and feel invincible, you may have an immediate family history of the disease; you might be a smoker; you might carry extra weight or have diabetes or high blood pressure or too much bad cholesterol. These are all dangers for developing heart disease. Yet it becomes *more* dangerous when awareness of the risks is lagging. It's rare to meet women under the age of 40 who acknowledge that the biggest threat to their health is heart disease. To be honest, women *over* 40 may not realize they are in jeopardy either. We often register a greater awareness of the so-called women's diseases, such as breast or ovarian cancer.

I'm determined to help set the record straight. In cardiac care, it's important to think of women as being equally as important as men. They not only are susceptible to the same risk factors but also have similar heart attack symptoms and benefit from the same tests, treatments and cardiac education and rehabilitation programs. But sadly, as studies show, women may not get the same level of care and attention that men do. We do not fully know why this is the case, although we will explore some of the contributing factors in the next few pages.

❤ **You need to know: Men tend to develop heart disease earlier in life than women. Otherwise, men and women are very similar in terms of symptoms, response to treatments and recovery.**

For the bigger picture, let's look at the statistical trends. In the time since my grandfather Ben passed away after a heart attack in the early 1970s, the death rates for cardiovascular illness have decreased in men. This is in large part due to public awareness and advances in care. In the last 40 years, cardiac health has benefited from new procedures and more effective and well-tolerated medications. In North America, we've also become much more attuned to the benefits of heart-healthy lifestyles. Most of us at least recognize the positive consequences of eating well and incorporating activity into our daily routines.

It's troubling, then, that more women today are dying of heart disease than ever before. It's not entirely clear why, but we know it's not just because the population is aging. According to the Heart and Stroke Foundation, by 2003 the number of deaths due to cardiovascular disease had become essentially equal in Canadian men and women. Over the last 30 years, heart disease has become an equal opportunity killer, period.[1]

It's important for you to understand the issues related to women and heart disease, whether you are a woman or have a woman in your life—a mother, a sister, a partner. We need to talk about the myths, the medicine and the dangers of denial. Here are some other common comments and questions I've tackled over the years.

"Why are the death rates from cardiovascular disease in women increasing?"

Let me preface my answer with two particularly relevant patient stories. A woman came to see me in my practice at St. Michael's Hospital in Toronto for a second opinion. She was 44 years old, married with two children and had a family history of heart disease. She'd woken up in the middle of the night with a heaviness in her chest. Short of breath, she turned to her husband and asked what to do. Because he had some understanding that women can have heart problems just as men do, he immediately said, "This might be your heart. Let's call 9-1-1 and get to the hospital." They did. Doctors quickly discovered she'd had a heart attack. She got the treatment she needed. She received an angioplasty, a minimally invasive procedure where you open up a blocked coronary artery. (We'll explain this more in Chapter 10.) She was subsequently given medications and completed a cardiac rehab program. The moral of the story is: Because she and her husband acted quickly and without hesitation, they got to the ER in time, before there was any significant, irreparable muscle damage in her heart. In the days and weeks that followed, she made a great recovery. She was given excellent care and did well.

Now compare her experience with that of a 64-year-old woman who came to my office. For more than a year, this busy, socially vibrant woman had been in the thick of planning a major charity event. Any large-scale project like this one comes with a long list of to-dos and expectations. On the day of the event, she began experiencing nausea and what felt like indigestion. But she remained committed to the night. Even as her symptoms worsened, she soldiered on, determined not to ruin her big night. Finally, as the party was in full swing and her discomfort became unbearable, she gave up and went home. For three days that followed, she and her husband discussed what had happened and debated what to do next. At no point did they link her symptoms to heart disease. By the time she sought treatment—for what was, in retrospect, a heart attack—she had already suffered moderate damage to her heart muscle. Because she waited so long to seek help, her recovery was more involved than that of the 44-year-old woman who didn't hesitate, and her heart muscle was damaged for the rest of her life. In many ways, she was lucky it wasn't worse.

The second story is a classic case of a woman—and it happens to men, too—who downplays or virtually ignores her pain in order to get on with the immediate job at hand, which is usually in service of others. When a woman reacts this way, it's as if she's saying, "There are more important things in life than *me.*" This mindset might explain why, statistically, a woman's risk of dying following a heart attack or stroke is significantly higher than a man's. Studies show that women are less likely to seek medical help in time. In the last decade, the Heart and Stroke Foundation's Heart Truth campaign (for which I was on the leadership council) compiled a survey on women and awareness. Only one in eight women surveyed understood that heart disease is her most serious health concern. Only one in three knew it is the leading cause of death. Half of the surveyed men and almost one-third of the women falsely believed that death rates for women are lower than those of men.

There may also be a difference in the care some women receive. Women are not as likely as men to be treated by a cardiovascular specialist, and they're not as likely to be transferred to a cardiac facility if they're at a smaller hospital without a specialty cardiac care unit.[2] Women are also less likely to have specialized tests and procedures—such as cardiac catheterization and revascularization of the arteries, with either angioplasty or bypass surgery (see Chapter 10).

❤ **You need to know: Studies suggest many Canadian women are unaware that heart disease is the leading threat to their health.**

"Do women really think that heart disease can't happen to them?"

I treat many women in my practice and have met hundreds who never imagined they might be susceptible to a heart attack or stroke until they had one. To some extent, that's understandable. Preventing cardiovascular disease is largely about what you can't feel or see. No ordinary person is able to "see" that plaque might be collecting in her arteries. You also can't see high blood pressure. You can't feel the cholesterol that increases the accumulation of plaque and can lead to heart attack and stroke. These diseases can often progress to a danger point well before you feel any symptoms. This makes it possible to ignore your risk factors, especially if you are of the opinion that your health is something to "fix" only when something goes wrong. Unfortunately, many people extrapolate that feeling fine is an excuse to indulge in unhealthy behaviours.

> The symbol for women and heart disease is the red dress. Both the American Heart Association's Go Red for Women campaign and the Canadian Heart and Stroke Foundation's Heart Truth campaign are designed to raise awareness of this important issue. For more information visit *www.goredforwomen.org* or *www.theheartruth.ca*.

That's the physical side, but there's also the social side. At the risk of generalizing, I'll say that women are socialized differently than men. Men tend not to hesitate when a doctor is advising them. Women are more contemplative, perhaps a little more innately skeptical. For instance, when I explain to a male patient that he needs a procedure such as an angiogram, he'll say, "Okay, Doc, whatever you say." When I present a woman with the same information, she will often have questions and need to think about it.

Since heart attacks are largely seen as a male phenomenon, men tend to be more aware of the symptoms than women. Many men will experience a feeling of unusual tightness or heaviness in the chest and, right away, they'll connect it to the heart. Now, it's true that a man could conceivably go to the emergency room with heartburn and think he's having a heart attack. That's not such a terrible approach. It's the second-guessing that impedes our care. In fact, I encourage you not to think twice about seeking medical help when you are feeling chest pain, whether it goes away when you rest or not. (You'll get to know these symptoms better in Chapter 5.)

Many women I know—women I see in my practice—prefer to be "troopers" with pain, an approach that is rarely advantageous. A busy woman tends to be in a perpetual whirlwind of activity. In aid of her family, friends and career demands, she will pack in an inordinate amount of time answering emails, running errands, meeting deadlines and organizing the domestic realm in any given day. She will say, "Someone has to get it all done"—and she does. As a woman, I understand this mentality implicitly. As a doctor, I'm more supportive of slowing down. Devote a bit of that considerable energy to taking care of yourself.

We all know that women are intensely proactive when it comes to the health of their kids, their spouses and their aging parents. But their own heart health often falls off the radar. Many of my patients are women in their career-climbing and parenting years—the do-it-all women of our day. No matter how old they are, what background they come from and what challenges they face, these women share a kind of selflessness I truly feel isn't constructive. I might even say it's dangerous—dangerous for the woman, and dangerous for the message it sends to society. I'm not blaming women in the least, because I think how we got here has a lot to do with accepted social norms and the pressures on women, whether they're self-imposed or not, to be nurturers, workers, mothers, partners and all-purpose organizers. But it's now deeply concerning to me that many women would rather tick off the last five items on their to-do list than go to an emergency room when they need one most. That's what happens when we put ourselves last. We put our health last. If you talk to most women past the age of 25, the common refrain is "I'm just so busy." That usually means they're making time for everyone in their lives but themselves.

"What's wrong with being selfless?"

I call it the type E personality. You are everything to everyone but yourself. It's very common in women. Several years ago, I saw a patient in her 50s who is the primary caregiver in her family. Her husband is disabled, and she has relatively young children. One day, during a holiday weekend, she started experiencing chest pain. It felt like a squeezing and tightness, and it bothered her greatly as she performed her household tasks. Clearly something was not right with her health. However, instead of going to the emergency room, she began worrying about her son and his plans to see a fireworks display later that evening. To ensure her son's social life was in order, she called a girlfriend. The friend agreed to give the boy a ride to see the fireworks. Only *then* did my patient drive to the emergency room. I am not making this up. As scary as this sounds, it's a true story. When she told me what had happened, I looked at her, laughed nervously and said, "What is wrong with this story?" The consequences could have been disastrous for her. Fortunately, her chest pain was not coming from her heart. It was actually due to a severe spasm in her esophagus. But this could only be confirmed with a trip to the ER—which should have been her first priority.

If it results in ignoring your symptoms, selflessness can be self-defeating. If you consider it a rare luxury to take a walk around the block, to pack a healthy lunch a few times a week or to retreat from the computer screen once in a blue moon, then that has a direct and negative impact on your risk for developing coronary heart disease. I know and understand where you're coming from, but I also strongly feel you're overdue for a change.

I give women this direct advice: If you don't take the time to take care of yourself, you won't be around to take care of others. As they'll tell you on an airplane, put your oxygen mask on first, before you put one on others. Prioritize your well-being. When it comes to cardiovascular health, your behaviours have a direct impact on your risk factors. We know all about the perils of leading inactive lives and eating a diet rich in saturated fats. This behaviour puts us in direct risk of heart attack and stroke. It's the same principle with our social behaviour, and the way we diminish our own health needs relative to the health of our loved ones. Dealing with the potential of developing heart disease is about understanding your risk factors. Discuss your health with your doctor; investigate if you're a target for heart disease in the first place. From there, it's about being positive, proactive—and realistic.

"Can women reduce their risk by taking estrogen as they age?"

If it were only that easy! The link between estrogen loss in menopause and an increased risk of cardiovascular disease has women wondering about a quick fix. Many assume that estrogen and progesterone replacement therapy, now commonly known as hormone replacement therapy (HRT), is a way of turning back the clock and staving off heart attacks.

Let me be absolutely clear. You can't reverse time. There's no role for hormone replacement therapy in the prevention of heart disease and stroke. In fact, the risks of HRT, which include blood clots, heart attack and stroke, can seriously outweigh the benefits—perceived or real. Even if HRT is shown to prevent bone problems and osteoporosis, or makes you "feel" younger, there are other better preventive treatments for women. To be blunt, HRT should be used only for severe symptoms of menopause (such as the vasomotor symptoms—hot flashes and sweating). It should be used for the shortest duration of time (less than four years) and at the lowest possible dose.

Many of you might find certain medical acronyms confusing, especially if they start to change over time. For instance, HRT is now also known as HT (for hormone therapy). As a cardiologist interested in women's health, I'm amazed no one came up with a better abbreviation. In medicine, HT also stands for hypertension!

I'm reminded of one of my patients, an 83-year-old woman who came to me for a rhythm problem of the heart. She was in a wheelchair, but she had a great quality of life. She was the matriarch of a close-knit family and often came to see me with an entourage in tow. I found it endearing to watch her in action. She'd arrive in my office and start bossing her family members around. This patient was on HRT, and I wanted her to come off it. But she was deeply resistant. She loved the way her skin felt on HRT, she told me. My worry as a cardiologist was that she was a prime target for a blood clot, particularly given the fact that she was wheelchair bound and immobile. After much discussion, ultimately, she allowed me to boss *her* around, and we got her off the HRT, decreasing her risk of clotting.

Studies have assessed the benefits and risks of HRT. The Women's Health Initiative (WHI), published in the *New Eng-*

land Journal of Medicine in 2003, was the first large randomized control trial to look at HRT in women. A randomized control trial is the best way scientists can study a treatment. In this clinical experiment, study subjects are randomly assigned either to receive a drug or to receive a placebo (fake sugar pill) instead. The researchers won't know which subject is taking real medication so that the results can be evaluated without biases. The conclusion of the WHI was illuminating. It found that HRT offered no significant medical benefit. In fact, HRT showed a slight tendency to harm women.[3] Nearly 17,000 postmenopausal women aged 50 to 79 years participated in the study. Participants were randomly assigned to receive HRT (estrogen and progesterone) or a placebo. After five years, the study was stopped because it showed a small but increased risk of breast cancer in women receiving the HRT. There was also a slightly increased risk of heart attack and dying from heart disease, an increased risk of stroke and a two-fold increase in the risk of blood clots in the legs or lungs. The increased risks associated with HRT usually occurred in the first year of treatment. The WHI did show some benefit to women taking HRT, including a reduction in hip fractures and even colon cancer, but overall, this benefit did not balance the excess risk of heart attack, stroke and breast cancer. In the WHI, 100 women for every 10,000 taking HRT would experience an adverse event. Clearly, we shouldn't take a "preventive" therapy if it causes harm—that doesn't make sense to me.

According to other studies, women who already have heart disease and are on HRT encounter a slightly increased risk of recurrent heart attack or stroke.[4] The American Heart Association recommends that women stay off HRT for at least one year after a heart attack. That being said, women who also take adequate doses of cholesterol medication are less likely to have a heart attack or stroke—even if they are on HRT.

If you have heart disease and need to cope with *severe* symptoms of menopause, you might want to be on a low dose of HRT. The risk of HRT, in this case, is small and likely outweighed by the benefits—namely improving your quality of life. Talk to your doctor about it. As long as you are taking cholesterol-lowering medications for your heart disease and are aware of the risks and benefits, it might be reasonable to use HRT.[4]

And what about estrogen for men? Believe it or not, this is a question I get asked from time to time. The hypothesis is that if women are generally protected against heart attack and stroke until menopause, then giving estrogen to a man might reduce his risk as well. There's a mix of findings in this area. In a 1970 study called the Coronary Drug Project, men who were given estrogen after a heart attack had a higher risk of dying from blood clots in the lungs (or a pulmonary embolus).[5] More recently, the effects of estrogen have been studied in transgender individuals in Australia who were born male. In addition to growing breasts from this extreme intervention, men who received estrogen as part of gender reassignment saw beneficial effects on the function of their blood vessels. That being said, estrogen is not given to reduce risk of heart disease in men or women because of its other detrimental effects.

I have to be very direct with the women reading this, and with the men who love them. Changing the statistics related to women and heart disease starts with you. Be informed. Be proactive. Take charge of your health. You know the habits you have to break and the mindset you have to change. The question is, what are the specific steps you can take right now to promote heart-healthy living? The answers are next.

PART II

Preventing and Detecting Heart Disease

4

PRIMARY PREVENTION

"What can I do to protect myself and my family against heart disease?"

If you're facing any health crisis, especially one as potentially life altering—or life ending—as heart disease, then you might fall into thoughts of doom and gloom. I'm here to tell you that knowing you are at risk for heart disease is by no means a death sentence. Quite the opposite. There's a lot of good news on your side: You have access to a sophisticated health care system, with new advances in medicine every day. You also need little more than information and determination to meet your personal goals for reducing your risk. What I mean is, it doesn't take a modern piece of exercise equipment or an endless bank account to make a positive change for yourself or your family. Ironically, in this high-tech world, it's the low-tech solutions that make a difference—namely, diet and exercise.

❤ **You need to know: Studies show up to 80% of heart disease is preventable if you stop smoking, eat healthily, become active and form other long-lasting heart-healthy habits.**[1]

Still, society remains torn between virtue and indulgence. According to the latest research, the patterns of heart disease are changing because our attitudes are changing. On the one hand, we are seeing a reduction in high cholesterol, high blood pressure and smoking in the general population. All told, this accounts for about half of the reduction in coronary heart disease deaths. On the other hand, the same population is becoming more overweight and out of shape. Rates of obesity are soaring in North America. If this trend continues, we will reverse the good we've accomplished. With obesity comes high blood pressure, high cholesterol, diabetes and, of course, an increased risk for developing coronary heart disease.

There's no quick fix, magic bullet or high-tech miracle when it comes to prevention. The best way to protect yourself and your loved ones is to incorporate heart-healthy approaches into your life for the long term—before you develop heart disease. This is called primary prevention. I promise you: That's not the hardest thing in the world to achieve.

Here are the major areas to tackle.

Quit Smoking

This is, without a doubt, the single most important preventive intervention you can perform. Smoking is the leading preventable cause of disease, disability and death in Canada and throughout the world. The statistics here are staggering but, at the same time, not surprising: Half of regular smokers will die prematurely of smoking-related illnesses.

If you are a smoker, or if you have a family member or friend who is a smoker, you're probably well aware that tobacco is terrible for your health. If you are facing the prospect of quitting, you need a supportive approach to help you get over your addiction. If you smoke and wish to stop, remember to seek help, whether it's the support of your doctor or your family or both. Your doctor may encourage you to take medications as well. If you use nicotine replacements such as the patch, gum and inhalers as aids to quitting smoking, that's much less harmful than smoking itself.

❤ **You need to know: Smoking is the leading preventable cause of disease, disability and death in the country. But there's hope: Many smokers have the desire to quit and will respond to a supportive approach to breaking the habit.**

Although the amount of poison in each cigarette is small, its ongoing toxic effects in the body increase with each puff. Smoking is a tenacious addiction. Nicotine increases a hormone in the brain called dopamine, which gives you feelings of pleasure and calmness—levels that drop between cigarettes, leading to withdrawal symptoms such as irritability and stress. The more people smoke to avoid these withdrawal symptoms, the more nicotine they need to hit that level of pleasure and calm. What's more, when you puff a cigarette, the blood vessels constrict. This is the exact opposite effect of nitroglycerine, a drug we use in cardiac care. You may know this medication from being treated in the ER for chest pain related to your heart. When sprayed in the mouth, nitroglycerine offers quick relief of coronary chest pain by opening up, or dilating, the arteries. Smoking does the reverse: It closes your blood vessels.

If you quit smoking when you are younger than 40 years of age, you gain 9 years of life expectancy. If you quit when you are under 50 years old, you can gain 6 years of life expectancy. If you manage to quit while you are under 60, you can gain 3 years of life. If you quit when you are past retirement age, you will likely live longer than if you continued to smoke cigarettes. More importantly, you will improve your quality of life by reducing your chances of developing smoking-related disabilities such as chronic obstructive pulmonary disease (COPD) and emphysema.

Just as boys and girls start smoking for different reasons, men and women will quit for different reasons. Many women, for instance, are able to quit smoking during pregnancy. Amazingly enough, however, some women start up again when their children are older. They might even consider smoking a "grown-up time out." It may be easy to lapse back into smoking for a variety of reasons, but the benefits of quitting can't be overstated.

Within a year of giving up cigarettes, you are 50% less likely to develop coronary heart disease, compared with smokers.[2] Within 5 years, your risk of having a stroke returns to the same level as a non-smoker. (In contrast, your lung cancer risk unfortunately takes time to come down. Within 10 years of quitting smoking, the cancer risk is 50% less than your friends or family members who continue to smoke.) The encouraging news is that 15 years after quitting, your risk for cardiovascular disease is similar to peers who *never* smoked.

If you're a smoker, you may not consider your doctor someone who can truly motivate you to quit. Physicians are partially at fault when it comes to patients continuing to smoke. Doctors often find it frustrating to invest time in smoking counselling. They might spend the effort on the process, only to have the smoker fail in his attempts to quit. It's much easier for a doctor to prescribe a blood pressure medication—because a positive outcome is more predictable. Also, many doctors have not been trained properly on how to advise on smoking cessation.

When people initially quit smoking, they may have a worsening smoker's cough or sputum. This is because the lungs are essentially trying to get rid of all the toxins and—pardon the expression—crap that has built up over the years from smoking. It's a good thing!

As with all health matters, my advice to you is to be proactive. Studies suggest it's the personal rewards (as opposed to the health benefits) that motivate people to quit. If you are thinking about stopping, reflect on the gains that lie ahead. For instance, look at the money you'll save. If you have a smoking habit, you are probably spending thousands of dollars a year on cigarettes. Now, look closely at your parents, your children, your friends. Set a goal for smoking cessation that involves a milestone that's important to you and your family. For example, you might want to be smoke free and healthy at your son's graduation next summer or your niece's upcoming wedding. Think of the sense of accomplishment you'll feel and the life-changing health benefits that await you.

❤ **You need to know: If you have a family member or friend who smokes and you really want her to quit, it's helpful to discuss the non-health benefits of quitting, such as how much money she'll save or how much better her physical appearance will be.**

It can take some people many attempts to become smoke free, but quitting smoking is a process, not an event. Most data suggest that smokers who make multiple attempts to quit will eventually succeed.

You may be hesitant about taking cessation drugs. For example, you might feel the medication is too expensive (never mind how much money you'll save by not buying cigarettes in the long term). It's always amazed me that many drug insurance plans usually do not cover nicotine replacement or similar drugs. Smoking is a serious health issue!

Rest assured that the drugs work. According to the results of clinical trials, smokers on nicotine replacement patches and the

You should ask your doctor about any recent studies that have been conducted on the smoking-cessation medications on the market. For instance, in 2010, the Food and Drug Administration in the United States posted a safety communication concerning the use of varenicline in patients with cardiovascular disease. The FDA warned that the drug may be associated with a small increased risk of certain cardiovascular problems in patients who have heart disease. But from the perspective of many experts, and physicians who are helping their patients quit, this was an exaggeration of the results. In fact, the authors of the research stood by the safety of the drug, saying the study should reassure physicians of the safety of prescribing varenicline for smokers with stable heart disease.

smoking-cessation drug bupropion (known by the trade names Wellbutrin and Zyban) were almost twice as likely to quit as those not taking any medications. However, you have to realize there are differences between one cessation medication and the next. A medication like varenicline, for instance, works by blocking the nicotine receptor as well as releasing some amounts of dopamine. If you take varenicline (the trade name is Champix), you are less likely to have "excess pleasure" from sneaking a cigarette—because it blocks the effect of cigarettes. It is not the same case for nicotine replacements. If you try to smoke a cigarette while on the patch or chewing nicotine gum, you will feel an additional release of dopamine because the receptor is not blocked. Therefore, you may be more likely to start smoking again.

Varenicline originally received bad press for concerns that patients became depressed, moody and even suicidal while on the drug. However, looking at the data carefully, there's little evidence to support these claims. You have to keep in mind that when you are quitting smoking, your mood changes. If you are irritable, down or agitated, it is very important to talk to your doctor. In fact, the most common side effect of varenicline is nausea, which I tell my patients to overcome by drinking large amounts (eight large glasses) of water per day.

I will add that if you are living with coronary heart disease, you have to be cautious in taking smoking-cessation drugs. Your doctor will have some safety concerns if you go on these drugs. For instance, I would worry about your blood pressure on a drug such as bupropion.[3] On the other hand, varenicline has been proven effective in outpatients with coronary heart disease—it is reasonably safe.[4]

Eat Right

After quitting smoking, one of the key steps to take in the right direction of heart health is to eat nutritiously and in proper portion sizes. To prevent heart disease, and a host of other diseases, you benefit greatly from eating sensibly. One important point to acknowledge is there is no one particular food, vitamin or magic potion you can take to prevent heart disease that will serve you better than eating a healthy, balanced diet.

Good nutrition has a profound influence on our bodies. When I first started out in medicine, I was somewhat skeptical about just how much you can achieve with "natural" approaches to health and prevention. However, the older (and wiser) I get, the more I believe in the powers of healthy eating. A balanced diet that's low in saturated fats and high in fresh fruits and vegetables will set anyone in the right direction when it comes to protecting against heart disease.

When I stop to think about it, I've always been in the habit of eating healthily—thanks to my very determined and, frankly, avant-garde parents. My cardiologist dad was into heart-healthy behaviour in the 1970s, way before the rest of the world. He was also cholesterol crazy before it became trendy and incredibly strict when it came to avoiding fat in his diet. My mom often had to fib to him about how much butter or how many eggs she used to bake a cake. (I think she still does this to this day.) My father is a very well-balanced and kind person, but he would get frustrated with obese patients because he knew how much they were at risk.

At home, we practised what he preached. We were the only family I knew who went home for dinner and ate a main course called Monster Salad. It was basically a big leafy salad with lots of protein: eggs, chicken, turkey. We had it twice a week. My brother and I took healthy tuna-salad sandwiches to school, or half a bell pepper stuffed with low-fat protein. I remember when I was young, my best friend thought I was the craziest kid on the street because I'd take the skin off the Kentucky Fried Chicken and give it to her. What can I say? I was brainwashed as a young child.

Teaching your kids to be proactive about their health, including making healthy food choices, is one of the most important things you can do as a parent. I see it in young family members who shun the thought of eating fried chicken fingers because they have been taught since a young age to eat in a healthy way. Every one of us has time pressures, so it's a matter of making smart choices on the go: If you can pack a turkey sandwich for lunch and take it with you, that's great. If you're at a food court in the mall, a veggie-and-skim-cheese submarine sandwich with little (or no) dressing may be the best option around. Whatever you do, don't get anything fried or laden with saturated fats and sugar.

Thirty years later, I know that many parents invest a lot of effort into teaching their kids the same principles. My niece and nephew are now in the habit of eating fresh, nutrient-rich meals because their parents lead by example, just as my parents did. The trick for the rest of us grown-ups is to eat as well as these kids do! When you have no time and your calendar is full of meetings, that's not always easy.

My advice: First, know the keys to healthy eating and portion control. Second, focus on the healthy choices, but give yourself a little break once in a while, because most things are okay in moderation. Except, of course, cigarettes.

Many of us could benefit from talking to a dietitian about what exactly we are eating. You can ask your family doctor for a referral; it may even be covered under your health plan. Start with this 10-second questionnaire that I ask all my patients:

- Do you eat fried food?
- Do you leave the skin on chicken?
- Do you eat red meat more than once a month?
- Do you eat rich cheese?

If you have answered yes to these questions, it's very important that you read on. Here are the nine guideposts on the path to good nutrition.

Balance the four food groups. The Heart and Stroke Foundation recommends that you follow Canada's Food Guide, which means eating a balance of vegetables and fruit; breads and grains; milk and alternatives; and meats and alternatives. You can download a copy of this easy-to-use information sheet from Health Canada's website at www.hc-sc.gc.ca (look under Food and Nutrition) or get a copy sent to you by calling 1-800-OCANADA. The number of daily servings from each group depends on your age and gender.

For instance, Canada's Food Guide advises that if you're a woman between the ages of 19 and 50, you should aim to eat 7 or 8 portions of vegetables and fruit a day, 6 or 7 portions of grain products, 2 low-fat milk portions (or alternatives, like soy), and 2 portions of meat or protein alternatives.

In contrast, if you are a woman who is over the age of 50, or entering the menopausal years, you should eat 7 portions of vegetables and fruit a day, 6 portions of grains, 3 of milk or alternatives, and 2 portions of meat or protein alternatives.

Men aged 19 to 50 generally need more calories and nutrients from vegetables, whole grains and protein. The Food Guide advises they aim for 8 to 10 portions of vegetables and fruit a day, 8 portions of grains, 2 milk portions or alternatives, like soy, and 3 portions of meat or protein alternatives.

Men age 51 and over need 7 portions of vegetables and fruit a day, 7 of grains, 3 of milk, and 3 of meat or protein alternatives.

Fresh produce is a key to good nutrition. Eating 5 to 10 servings of vegetables and fruits a day will reduce your risk of heart attack and stroke. Most vegetables are low in calories, high in fibre (which helps fill you up) and rich in potassium and magnesium, which may help prevent plaque from narrowing your arteries. Specifically, potassium and magnesium help keep the electrical system working properly, the heart rhythm steady and blood pressure under control. And when it comes to breads and grains, look for *whole grain* on food packages. Make at least half of your grain servings whole grain every day. Eat a variety of grains such as brown rice, barley, oats and quinoa.

If you are uncertain about what a "serving" means, use these rules of thumb:

- For vegetables and fruit, one serving is one medium whole fruit (like an apple, a banana or an ear of corn). Or generally, 1/2 cup of any chopped vegetable or fruit is considered one serving. The exception is most leafy greens such as mesclun salad mix or spinach. One serving size of these is equal to 1 cup.
- For grains, one serving is either a slice of bread (35 grams) or 30 grams of cereal or 1/2 cup of cooked pasta or rice.
- For dairy and alternatives, one serving is either 1 cup

of milk, 3/4 cup of yogurt or 1.5 ounces (50 grams) of cheese such as cheddar, feta or mozzarella.
- For meats and proteins, one serving is either 2 eggs or 3/4 cup of beans and legumes, or the equivalent of 1/2 cup (or small fist-sized) portion of beef, chicken, fish, turkey and so on.

Drink water. Canada's Food Guide also advises that you drink fluids regularly. Try to satisfy your thirst with water; it should be your first choice of drink. Tap water will do! Limit your intake of soft drinks, caffeinated beverages, fruit juices, energy drinks and alcohol. These tend to be high in calories, or low in nutrients, or both. Switching from soda pop and juices to plain water will help you lower calorie and sugar intake and keep you hydrated.

I have a close friend who's a nutritionist. Her brother, who lives in England, asked her for advice on how to get into shape. Amazingly, she was able to help him lose 26 pounds in six months—a healthy rate of one pound a week—by following her three rules of nutritious eating. Her first rule: Don't drink your calories. Second: Eat healthy, non-processed foods. Finally, she told her brother to get his butt off the couch and start exercising. With all the pubs and fried food in England, losing weight was a challenge. But he did it.

❤ **You need to know: Substituting water for soda pop and juices is one small step to leading a healthier life.**

Prepare right-sized portions of healthy foods in advance. As with many things besides food, when your consumption gets out of control, you suffer. We're living in a toxic environment with unhealthy food options everywhere around us. It's the era of "super sizing." If you actually look at the calorie count in food today, compared with many years ago, portions are bigger and there are more fat and calories in processed and takeout food. According to recent American studies, over the past 30 years the average total calories taken in by American adults alone increased by 22% in women and 10% in men. This reflects a larger intake of carbohydrates, larger portion sizes and increased consumption of snacks, fast-food meals and sugar-sweetened beverages such as pop.[5] As a consequence, we are seeing more risk factors for heart disease in young adults.[6]

Our societal expectations have also radically changed. Just recall the last time you went into a restaurant and were served a small portion. You probably thought, "Wow, that's so tiny, I'm not getting my money's worth," instead of accepting the fact that this is a healthier size meal to consume.

> The toxic food environment is an international problem. In India, for instance, modernization has led to increasing rates of obesity and risk of heart disease. Men, women and children are leading less of what's called a healthy rural life and more of an unhealthy urban life—they walk less, use cars more and have moved away from consuming a traditional, healthier diet based on vegetables and grains.

A more sensible approach to eating is to think of how much food you *need* and devote a little time to preparing your portions in advance. I am a 5-foot-tall woman who can eat only so much during the day. To maintain my weight, I need to consume about 1,500 calories daily. I don't need as many calories as my 6-foot-3 husband, to say the least. One handy trick I adopted years ago is to spend an hour each week cooking a big batch of chicken breasts, turkey and fish fillets, which I put in small Tupperware containers (each holds about 4 ounces of protein) and freeze. Every morning, I take one out and bring it to work with me. I call it the surprise lunch because I don't know exactly what is inside. I also bring a baggie of cut-up vegetables, an apple or orange and water, and sometimes low-fat cheese sticks and Melba toast. The first thing I do when I get home at the end of the day, no joke, is to chop vegetables and make a big salad, usually with the TV or radio on in the background. It's a small investment in time that results in a large payoff in my health.

Of course, I love food and enjoy eating out, but if I ate out daily, even if I were watching myself, I would gain weight without blinking. I bring my lunch to work and prepare foods so I can enjoy going out when I want, without feeling guilty. When you're eating out, you know that restaurant portions can be too large. One good trick is to order an appetizer as a main course.

Most people I ask who are overweight say they don't eat a lot, which frankly is not usually true. It reminds me of a politically incorrect story I heard involving an insensitive physician and a patient in denial. A woman weighing close to 300 pounds had just had a heart attack and was sitting in bed in the coronary care unit. A senior physician wanted to try to approach her about weight loss. She said to him, "Doctor, I swear I eat like a bird." His response was, "Well, if you eat like a bird, it must be a pterodactyl." He must have had some people skills because she didn't take offence. . . . Old-school medicine, I guess.

Read the labels on food packaging. Pick up two items off the shelf at the grocery store. If one has more fat or more calories, put that item down. Reading supermarket packaging gives you an important snapshot of what's in the food you're eating. As the Heart and Stroke Foundation advises, it's important to know that the ingredients on food labels are listed in descending order by weight. This means the higher the ingredient is on the list, the greater the amount in the food. If your first ingredient is sugar or fat, just put the box back on the shelf. Fats can be listed as lard, shortening, oils (palm, coconut, hydrogenated), monoglycerides, triglycerides or talo. Sugars can be listed as honey, molasses, syrups or anything that ends in *ose* (dextrose, sucrose, fructose, maltose, lactose). Salt is another tricky one on food labels. MSG, sodium, brine and soya sauce are synonymous with salt. If you have a tendency for high blood pressure or a family history of high blood pressure, watch the salt in your diet.

The other key part of the label is the nutrition facts table, which details the nutritional content per serving. But be careful here. Remember to take note of the serving size. If there are only 50 calories per serving but the item you are looking at adds up to five servings per package, then you could easily be taking in 250 calories for a snack food you might have considered low calorie.

Be aware of fat—and stick to low-fat foods. We live in a world where there are hidden fats and calories in most foods, especially ready-made options in grocery stores and restaurants. Too much fat intake can increase our bad cholesterol (LDL) and pack on the pounds, which might lead to hypertension and promote the buildup of plaque in our arteries.

Choose the low-fat options of dairy and alternatives, such as low-fat milk, cheese, yogurt or fortified soy beverages. These are an important source of calcium and other nutrients. I have many cheese lovers in my practice who have been able to lower their cholesterol just by switching to lower-fat cheese. For some, however, indulging in cheese is practically an addiction. One of my patients is a bright, middle-aged man who was very overweight and out of shape and had developed diabetes. For some time, he kept a secret from me: He was eating a pound of cheese a day. Ultimately, the truth came out, and with great determination, the patient made a series of crucial lifestyle changes. As soon as he left the cheese habit behind, he started losing a great deal of weight. His diabetes improved. His hypertension became more controlled, and I decreased his blood pressure medication. He was able to lose nearly 100 pounds and keep it off with healthy eating and eliminating the higher-fat, higher-calorie cheese in his diet. He still needed cholesterol medication because he had had a heart attack. However, cholesterol pills will not work in isolation.

You need to take them while maintaining a low-fat diet. In the end, he reduced his risk of future heart problems.

In my diet, I opt for healthier meats and sources of protein. I prefer to get my iron from turkey, which is lower in fat than beef, and from shrimp. Chicken, lean beef, fish, beans, nuts and soy products are all good sources of protein that satisfy your hunger and are lower in fat. I personally eat very little red meat—only once a month!—but eat lots of turkey, fish and chicken. Skin off, of course.

Although it's impractical to eliminate fats completely from our diets, you must choose them carefully and use only the best unsaturated fats in moderation. Unsaturated vegetable oils include olive, canola, corn, flaxseed and sunflower oil.

Health Canada advises that only 20% to 35% of your calories come from fat. This amounts to approximately three to five tablespoons of oil per day in women and four to six tablespoons for men.

Remember, there are all sorts of hidden fats in what you eat—part of the toxic environment of fast, greasy food all around us. To try to reduce your portions and intake, use reduced-fat products whenever possible such as skim milk and low-fat salad dressings.

In terms of fat, you consume three main types: unsaturated, saturated and trans fats. Unsaturated fats can help lower the LDL (bad) cholesterol. Saturated fats, however, worsen your cholesterol levels. Trans fats are the worst fats of all for your health.

There are two types of unsaturated fats: monounsaturated and polyunsaturated. Monounsaturated fats lower LDL cholesterol and are found in olive and canola oils and some soft, non-hydrogenated margarines. Polyunsaturated fats are either omega 3 or omega 6. Omega-3 fats help prevent blood from thickening and clotting and also help lower triglycerides, decreasing the risk of heart attack and stroke. This fat is found in fish such as salmon, mackerel, herring and sardines as well as in flax and newer products on the market such as omega-3 eggs. Omega 6 is liquid at room temperature and is found in sunflower, corn and sapphire oils; non-hydrogenated margarines; and almonds, pecans, brazil nuts, sunflower seeds and sesame seeds. Although omega 6 can help lower LDL (bad) cholesterol, too much of it is a bad thing. When eaten in large amounts, it can also lower the HDL (good) cholesterol. Canadian diets tend to be high in amounts of omega 6.

Saturated fats are solid at room temperature and generally come from meat, poultry and dairy products. Plant sources of saturated fat are coconut oil, palm oil and palm kernel oil. Since saturated fat can raise LDL cholesterol, reducing your intake is an important step in lowering your risk of heart disease and stroke. Choose lean meats, remove skin from chicken and consume lower-fat dairy products. In addition, use any cooking method that allows fat to drain off, such as broiling, grilling or roasting on a rack.

❤ **You need to know: Reducing your intake of saturated fat is key to lowering your risk of heart disease and stroke. Choose lean meats, skinless chicken and low-fat dairy products, and remember to broil, grill or roast meats on a rack, allowing the fat to run off.**

As for trans fats, just stay away from them! This fat is created when an unsaturated fat is processed, or hydrogenated. Like saturated fat, trans fat raises LDL (bad) cholesterol. It is found in some partially hydrogenated margarines as well as many crackers, cookies and commercially baked products (look for "partially hydrogenated" or "vegetable oil shortening" in the ingredients). It can also be found in deep-fried food from fast-food outlets.

As the Heart and Stroke Foundation advises, eliminating trans fats in packaged foods is important, but it will not necessarily make the food healthier. High sugar and salt content and overall number of calories are dangerous factors, too.

I once saw a patient in our hospital's Cardiac Prevention Centre who was 44, South Asian and recovering from a heart attack. In addition to cholesterol-lowering medications, we had advised him on heart-healthy eating, which included eating more whole grains. He vowed to follow the health care team's counsel. But we'd see him every few months in the clinic and were perplexed. His cholesterol kept rising when he swore he was taking his medication and eating the food we suggested. The mystery was finally solved when the dietitian asked his wife to come in and review what she had been cooking. It turned out he was eating more whole grains in the form of granola bars, as our dietitian had suggested. The only problem was that she was *frying* them—in coconut oil!

Focus on fresh sources of vitamins and nutrients rather than supplements. I'm a firm believer that we can obtain most of our daily intake of vitamins through good old-fashioned fruit and vegetables. Try to eat 8 to 10 servings of vegetables and fruit daily. Although that sounds like a lot, it really isn't. If you cut up vegetables or take a piece of fruit with you to work or as a snack at home, you are on the way to improving your heart health.

To obtain the most nutrients and the ideal number of calories, Canada's Food Guide advises that you do the following:

- Opt for vegetables and fruit prepared with no added fat, sugar and salt.
- Choose more fresh vegetables and fruit—instead of juice.
- Eat at least one dark green and one orange vegetable daily. Ideal vitamin-rich dark vegetables include broccoli, spinach and kale. Ideal orange vegetables include carrots, sweet potatoes and squash.
- Steam or bake your vegetables instead of frying them.

I'd love to believe that eating chocolate protects the heart. But sorry to say, this isn't proven. Yes, dark chocolate has fewer calories and a lower fat content than other chocolate. But despite many studies trying to find an association between chocolate and prevention of heart disease, the results are not conclusive. That being said, if you are a chocoholic—as I am—having a few squares or other sweets in your diet is not unreasonable. In moderation, it's fine. Just as long as you're eating sensibly otherwise and not gaining weight.

Also, omega-3 fatty acids and certain fish oils have been associated with protection against sudden death and heart disease. Eating fish twice per week will help reduce your risk.

Minimize your salt intake. Salt in your diet is associated with high blood pressure. The reasons are complex, but they're related to the fact that your salt intake is managed by your kidneys. When we consume too much sodium, our kidneys can't control the intake, and the salt ends up in our blood, attracting water. This causes our blood pressure to rise.

The Heart and Stroke Foundation recommends that you limit sodium consumption. To reduce added, unnecessary salt,

- cut down on prepared and processed foods;
- look for products with claims such as low sodium, sodium reduced or no salt added;
- eat more fresh vegetables and fruit;
- reduce the amount of salt you add while cooking, baking or at the table;
- experiment with other seasonings, such as garlic, lemon juice and fresh or dried herbs;
- when eating out, ask for nutrient information for the menu items, and select meals lower in sodium; and
- look for the Health Check symbol on foods. Health Check is the Heart and Stroke Foundation's food information program, based on Canada's Food Guide.

Canadians actually consume a lot more sodium than we realize, at an average of 3,400 mg of salt per person, per day. If you have heart disease, we recommend you take in less than 1,500 mg of salt. So consider this when you look at the sodium values on food packaging.

A few more tips on reducing salt intake: Remove the salt shaker from your dinner table. Out of sight, out of mind. Also, choose fresh and frozen foods instead of canned or bottled goods; salt is a preservative in non-perishable items. Avoid processed foods such as deli meats, dry soup mixes, casserole mixes, smoked meat and fish, salted nuts and potato chips. When cooking, instead of salt, use fresh or dried herbs, lemon juice, flavoured vinegar and spices such as curry, paprika or ginger. Understand that many restaurants, fast food or otherwise, pile on the salt because they think it will appeal more to customers. Certain foods—soups, dipping sauces, Asian cuisine that uses soy sauce—can be astronomically high in salt.

I do believe you can train your taste buds. Once you limit the salt at home, you'll begin to taste it when you eat out. And after a while, that non-homemade food will taste overly salty. I instruct my patients who have congestive heart failure (see Chapter 12) and are *not* allowed to add any salt to their meals to try eating foods with pepper or a distinctive spice or flavour they love, like cumin or ginger.

Be skeptical of fad foods. As a rule, I wouldn't jump on any food that's touted as the "next best thing." By that, I mean that every day there's a new and trendy antioxidant food or drink on the market. It may be pomegranate juice. It may be the açai berry. Many of these *are* good for you to consume. But there are lots of claims out there that taking in an increased amount of just one substance can lower your risk for having heart disease. On its own, nothing is a miracle worker. Especially not a supplement. You must remember that the vitamin and supplement market in

North America is a multi-billion-dollar for-profit industry. Every week, I see a new pitch for a new compound or supplement that has not been rigorously tested and proven to reduce heart disease. I caution my patients not to believe the hype. As for how to discern good information from bad, here's a rule of thumb: Look for approval from a large, well-respected organization such as the Heart and Stroke Foundation or the American Heart Association. In other words, if you see a commercial or magazine ad for a particular miracle "diet" or food, and it doesn't come with support from a credible organization, then buyer beware.

Look for the Health Check symbol. Grocery shopping for healthy foods can sometimes be complicated and time consuming. Eating out can also be fraught with challenges to eating in a heart-healthy manner. To help consumers quickly identify products that contribute to healthy, balanced diets, the Heart and Stroke Foundation created a not-for-profit food information program called Health Check. As part of the program, registered dietitians evaluate grocery products and menu items that voluntarily enter the program and must meet nutrient criteria based on recommendations in Canada's Food Guide. When the product has been approved, the manufacturer is allowed to use the Health Check symbol on the packaging. The Health Check symbol can be found on many foods including grain products, vegetables and fruits, milk and alternatives, and meat and alternatives. For more information, including additional nutrition tips and recipes, visit www.healthcheck.org.

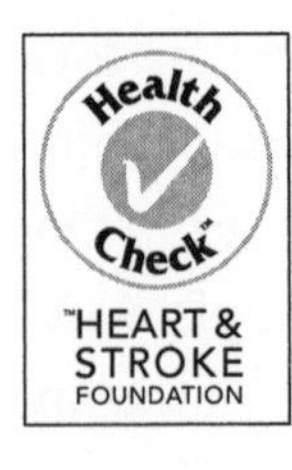

Get Active

Eating well goes hand in glove with an active approach to life. Exercise—whether you're walking briskly or working out on cardio equipment in a gym—help you burn calories and benefits your heart and blood vessels. Activity reduces your tendency for high blood pressure, high cholesterol and diabetes. It can also reduce C-reactive protein (CRP) levels, which is a marker for inflammation and is associated with heart disease (see Chapter 2). As your doctor will assure you, the best approach for overall health is to maintain good nutrition plus exercise. As my father used to always tell me, "Walking is good for the heart."

The Heart and Stroke Foundation recommends that adults be moderately or vigorously active for 30 to 60 minutes a day most days of the week. (From a realistic perspective, I tell my patients to try for 30 minutes of sweaty exercise, three times a week.) This includes walking, cycling, raking the leaves, swimming or dancing. The activity doesn't have to be done all at once. It can be added up in periods of at least 10 minutes over the course of a day. Children should be active, cumulatively, for at least 90 minutes a day most days of the week. More vigorous activities, such as going to an aerobics class, jogging, playing hockey or shooting hoops, can be engaging as well as rewarding, but they are not necessarily needed to maintain your heart health.

❤ **You need to know: You should engage in moderate to vigorous activity—so you are short of breath and sweaty—for 30 to 60 minutes, most days of the week.**

Here are other guidelines to consider. Recently, both Health Canada and the Canadian Society for Exercise Physiology (CSEP) have changed their recommendations on healthy lifestyles and regular activity so that the goals are more achievable. CSEP now

Where you live has an impact on your health. In the suburbs, the "built environment" may not be as conducive to activity and good health. It's easier for you to get into a car and drive to your nearest big-box store and amenities rather than walk to shop. This is why there is a fallacy about living in a big city. Cities are associated with unhealthy lifestyles. However, it can actually be healthier to live in urban centres if you can walk where you need to go.

recommends 60 minutes of activity per day for children, and 2.5 hours weekly for adults instead of 7 hours, as previously recommended.[7] It's not that *more* activity isn't good for you. It's just that in our jam-packed lives, reasonable and achievable goals make more sense. The important take-home point is that we should all embrace a regular, scheduled pattern of activity, regardless of our age or stage in life.

A good place to begin getting active is within the family. Children of active parents are more likely to participate in physical activity and also more likely to continue being more active as they grow. You can start with as simple a routine as participating in a nightly neighbourhood walk with your children or spouse. Try to minimize using the car for small shopping errands. Your walking will increase, and your health will benefit from it. We have to stop the "circle the mall for the closest parking space" mentality.

What is the specific impact on your heart? To begin with, physical activity helps make your heart and cardiovascular system strong and healthy. Regular exercise can, in fact, lower your blood pressure and therefore help prevent heart disease and stroke. As we covered in Chapter 2, blood pressure is the force exerted on the walls of the arteries by the blood as your heart pumps. Think about the analogy of a garden hose, where the water is turned up too high and the pressure ends up being too strong. The water will end up wrecking your flower beds. If your blood pressure becomes elevated, and the force exerted on the artery walls is too much, then that's not good for your heart. A consequence of high blood pressure is that, over time, it can cause your heart muscle to thicken. It can also increase your risk for developing atherosclerosis.

If you exercise on a regular basis, your heart and blood vessels become healthier. Exercise can help you maintain a healthy weight and even prevents your blood pressure from rising as you get older. The key is to be active not just once or twice a year, but to conduct an active lifestyle so you can achieve sustainable results. Many studies show that if you are active, you will live a longer, healthier life.

> To combat the epidemic of youth obesity, and to engender heart-healthy behaviour from the earliest ages, the Heart and Stroke Foundation recommends children incorporate daily physical activity into their routines. If your kids are not getting enough fresh air and running around during the school day, especially in the winter, talk to their educators. Create an active schedule after school; it's important to find time for play or activity outdoors as a family. Balance is, of course, key. If your children are spending all their free time on homework obligations or after-school academic activities, focus on liberating them for a little more outdoor play time.

Activity can also help reduce high cholesterol and high blood sugars. It can reduce the risk of second or third heart attacks in patients living with heart disease. In addition, activity has been shown to help significantly in our psychological well-being and reduce rates of depression. Studies have shown a relationship between sedentary activities (such as using a computer, playing video games, watching television and reading) and overall physical inactivity. According to the research, the more time people spend commuting to and from work in a car, the less likely they are to be physically active and the more likely they are to be overweight or obese. It speaks to our busy lives. If you are commuting, you need to schedule activity into your lifestyle.

Incorporating some form of movement into your daily routine will likely be a more lasting lifestyle change than starting to exercise and joining a gym. That being said, I do ask my patients when they come into my office if they are "exercising" in the gym sense of the word, because quite often, we need patients to do both moderate activity and intentional exercise.

If you're averse to pulling on a pair of spandex tights and joining a gym, I understand. Walking briskly is a great place to begin. Pick up an inexpensive pedometer and measure your footsteps—adding up to 10,000 steps a day, whether they're brisk or moderately so, is terrific. The one device you won't need is a heart rate monitor, which measures how fast your heart is beating. Unless you have already been diagnosed with heart disease or are training for the Olympics, you don't need to monitor how high your heart rate goes. You will know you've reached an activity level that is high enough if you are short of breath and sweating.

Most of us need to schedule activity into our calendars, just as we would schedule a doctor's appointment, work meeting or dinner with friends. But there are some routines in which activity slips in naturally: If you take public transit to work, get off a few stops before your destination and walk. If you're like me and always running late to work, then leave the power walk for the way home at the end of the day. If you work in a building with elevators, take the stairs. If you shop for groceries, walk to the store.

Promise yourself you'll do this for a month straight, and soon the habits will start becoming ingrained in your daily life. Before long, you'll be bounding up flights of steps at the office, and you will probably drop a pant size or two.

Maintain a Healthy Body Weight

When it comes to weight loss, the math is simple. To lose weight, it's about calories in *minus* calories out. Most of us need to eat smaller, healthier portions of our daily meals, and we need to engage in regular activity. You don't need your doctor to advise you of the ideal weight range corresponding to your height. You can look it up online at the National Heart Lung and Blood Institute site at www.nhlbi.nih.gov/guidelines/obesity/bmi_tbl.htm. But remember it's not always a matter of pure numbers. You can be very thin and lack nutrition from an inadequate food intake—for example, if you eat fatty cheese and nothing else. A healthy body weight has nothing to do with being skinny. The goal is to be healthy on the inside, even if that means 5 to 10 pounds of extra weight on the outside.

Here are some basic goals to keep in mind.

Be honest about your weight. Not everyone needs to go on a calorie-restricted diet to lose weight. If you are slightly overweight, do not have a large waist and have fewer than two risk factors for heart disease (see Chapter 2), you may need to prevent further weight gain rather than *lose* weight. Just watch the "creep"—putting on a couple of pounds a year but not noticing it. This can add up, especially as your metabolism changes as you age. You may need to cut down on some of the caloric intake in your day-to-day routine as you get older just to maintain your weight.

By contrast, if you are slightly overweight but have an increased waist circumference (if you're carrying your weight on your belly) or two or more heart disease risk factors, your risk is similar to someone who is technically obese, which is having a body mass index over 30. In this case, losing 5% to 10% of your current weight can help lower future risk. (For more on waist circumference, see Chapter 2.)

Take a slow and steady approach to weight loss. When it comes to losing weight, no one diet is safer or better than another. The truth is, I don't believe in fad diets.

A recent study in the *New England Journal of Medicine*[8] looked at different types of diets to see which are more effective. Its conclusion was that it really didn't matter if you were eating low carb or not, as long as you were taking in fewer calories in a day. I do feel strongly, however, that you should never be eating high-fat foods. A carb-free, high-fat and high-protein diet is not in the least bit healthy.

Small, gradual changes in your behaviour such as cutting down portion size and adding healthier food choices ultimately will help you be healthier and maintain a healthier body weight. If you need to lose weight, doing it gradually and sustainably—0.5 to 1 pound a week—is always better than fast weight loss. A slower rate of weight loss means you're changing your lifestyle for the better and not going on a quick diet that you'll eventually abandon. When losing weight, being accountable to yourself and someone else is often useful. A ritual where you weigh in weekly, in front of a friend or family member or in a program, is often effective from a behavioural and motivational perspective.

> The most effective weight loss programs are the ones that suggest making small but sensible choices in your daily routine. The reason doctors don't recommend fad diets is that, although they may bring about very quick weight loss, you will usually gain back the weight because it's difficult to maintain severely calorie-reduced diets for the rest of your life. Instead, eat smaller portions, follow a nutritious meal plan, commit to physical activity and change your everyday routine for a long and lasting effect.

Set your goals for weight loss. Measure, monitor, plan and stick with it. Some of the most useful advice I've ever seen on weight loss comes from the National Heart Lung and Blood Institute (NHLBI), a division of the National Institutes of Health, located in Bethesda, Maryland. The organization recommends these excellent steps[9] to help you reach a healthy weight:

Determine your body mass index. You may recall from Chapter 2 that BMI—a measure of body fat and a good indicator of risks for heart disease—is equal to your weight divided by the square of your height. A BMI of less than 18.5 means you're underweight.

Normal weight is 18.5 to 24.9. Overweight is 25 to 29.9. Finally, obese is a BMI of more than 30.

Measure your waist circumference. If your fat is distributed around your waist, then you are at risk for heart disease and diabetes. The risk goes up with waist size that is generally greater than 88 cm (35 in.) for women and 102 cm (40 in.) for men; if you are Asian, South Asian or South or Central American, and your body type is generally smaller than that of Caucasians, the values are 80 cm (32 in.) for women and 90 cm (35 in.) for men. To correctly measure your waist, stand and place the tape measure around your middle just above your hip bones. Measure your waist just after you breathe out. Sorry, sucking in your tummy isn't going to give you the right answer!

Know your risk factors. Look back at Chapter 2 for a complete lowdown on the risks—high cholesterol, hypertension, family history of early heart disease, smoking, diabetes and physical inactivity. Combined with excess weight, these risks can be very dangerous.

Focus on lifestyle change. Most people trying to lose weight focus just on the goal of weight loss, without thinking about how to incorporate healthy eating and exercise routines for the rest of their lives. Making a lasting lifestyle change is most important.

Set realistic and useful goals. That is, try to be less than perfect. Walking 5 km every day is specific and measurable, but for most of us, it's not attainable. Walking 30 minutes day in and day out is more realistic. But what happens if you are held up at work or it rains during your walking time? Walking 30 minutes five days a week is specific, doable and forgiving.

The NHLBI also gives great tips for achieving your goals:

Make your goals short-term ones—and write them down. Move ahead in small steps. For example, you may wish to reduce your intake by 100 calories a day initially, then 300 and eventually 500 calories.

Monitor your weight. Regular weekly weigh-ins are essential to keep you honest and on track. It's about having a formal routine—you can even ask a family member to weigh you in. It's about being accountable to yourself and your goals; don't avoid the scale, which enables you to easily slide back into bad habits. I cannot tell you the number of patients that come through my office who are overweight, with heart disease or risk factors, who don't own a scale. It might seem obvious—but you have to measure your progress and write it down.

Keep a food diary. Holding to a detailed record of your daily food intake will help you stay on track when trying to lose weight or maintain a healthy weight. Printable food-diary forms can be downloaded from www.nhlbi.nih.gov.

Monitor your behaviour. You need to observe and record some aspects of your behaviour you weren't aware of before, along with the milestones you reach along the way. This may be the quantity of fruit and vegetables in your diet, the number of unhealthy fast-food meals you eat or the amount of physical activity you participate in. Self-monitoring allows you and those helping you to know how you're really doing.

Reward success. Celebrate even small milestones—but not with food! And don't tell yourself you're waiting until the end, *Biggest Loser*–style, to give yourself a big present.

In the end, achieving a healthy weight is nothing short of a praiseworthy accomplishment. I know that weight loss is difficult. When you're losing weight and changing your lifestyle, you may be dealing with some possibly long-neglected personal issues. It is helpful to lean on a support network to help you get through them. Enlist your friends and family to share your goals, to join you in healthy grocery shopping and to prepare and eat the same meals as you do. You want to feel positive and included, not deprived and excluded.

A recent study proves that even very obese individuals—those with a BMI of 43—can achieve sustainable weight-loss goals. Participants followed a simple regimen of reducing their caloric intake and progressively increasing physical activity. They built up to walking briskly for 60 minutes, five times per week—in 10-minute intervals. Study participants were given a pedometer and a goal of more than 10,000 steps per day. The individuals who lost 5% to 10% of their body weight saw a reduction in their blood pressure, cholesterol and diabetes.[10]

Manage Cholesterol—Good or Bad

Cholesterol in the body becomes elevated for two reasons—increased consumption of high-fat foods or genetics. Most of us can reduce our cholesterol levels by about 20% by changing our diets. People who don't have established heart disease may be able to control their cholesterol with diet and lifestyle changes alone.

However, all my patients living with coronary heart disease, stroke or peripheral arterial disease need to be on cholesterol medications *in addition to* watching what they eat. This is regardless of one's baseline cholesterol levels. Many large studies (called randomized controlled clinical trials; see Chapter 16) have shown the benefits of taking a cholesterol pill, specifically the class of drugs called statins, or Lipitor-type meds. These drugs reduce the level of LDL (bad) cholesterol in the blood, thereby reducing your risk of dying from heart disease, recurrent heart attack or stroke.

Many of you who take cholesterol medications are worried about side effects, specifically those of statins. But most heart medications have no side effects at all. A small percentage of patients may develop muscle aches when they start cholesterol pills, and there can be a mild abnormality in liver function tests. But these are the exceptions to the rule. These side effects are treatable, and they reverse when you stop the medications. If you started on a cholesterol pill, you should have your blood checked every 6 to 12 months (depending on your health history). The blood test is to assess liver function and muscle function. The muscle function (enzyme) blood test is called CK. Not all of my patients who have muscle aches actually have an abnormality in the muscle enzyme when taking these medications. If you have a muscle ache on one type of statin, then switching to another statin may not give you the same symptoms.

I'll emphasize that if you need cholesterol medication, you should take it. Statistics show that millions of people who need medications don't take them. Recent data from the United States suggest that fewer than half the people who qualify for any kind of cholesterol-modifying treatment to lower their risk for heart disease are receiving that drug, and fewer than half of the highest-risk patients—those living with coronary heart disease—are taking cholesterol drugs on an ongoing basis. This isn't because these drugs haven't been prescribed. In my experience, patients are leery about taking these medications even after I explain that these drugs, when needed, are safe and effective. If you are living with heart disease, or at risk, and your physician has written a prescription for medications, do yourself a favour—take the medication!

❤ **You need to know: If you are living with heart disease, fill your prescription for cholesterol medication. The pills will reduce your risk for future heart problems, even if your cholesterol is not that high.**

Besides taking your medication, you can make positive food choices to help manage your LDL and HDL levels. The Heart and Stroke Foundation has a great checklist of 10 simple ways to get your cholesterol under control.

In 2006, Canada's Trans Fat Task Force recommended legislation to limit trans fats in processed foods. A partnership between Health Canada and the Heart and Stroke Foundation, the task force called for trans fat to be limited to 2% of total fat content in spreadable margarine and 5% in all other foods. The following year, a report by Toronto Public Health called for the federal government's swift action to eliminate harmful trans fat in Canada. To date, certain municipalities, food manufacturers and restaurants are making progress—but trans fat is still present in a variety of consumer foods marketed to adults and children all over North America.

1. Reduce your fat intake to 20% to 35% of your daily calories. Reading labels is important. Put the item down if the fat content is high!
2. Choose healthy fats such as polyunsaturated and monounsaturated fats mainly found in vegetable oils, nuts and fish.
3. When eating fat, limit your intake of the saturated fat mainly found in red meat and high-fat dairy products. Cheese is a no-no that even my health-conscious patients forget (or at least pretend to forget, as they tend to be cheese lovers). Sticking to low-fat yogurts and skim milk can sometimes make all the difference in controlling your cholesterol.
4. Avoid trans fats in foods. They are toxic to our arteries.
5. Instead of fad diets, use Canada's Food Guide to plan a healthier diet. Essentially, eat more whole grains, cereals, vegetables and fruit. This will keep your cholesterol under better control.
6. Snack wisely. Choose low-salt pretzels, plain popcorn or fruit rather than higher-fat or junk food snacks.
7. Use broiling, steaming and other lower-fat cooking methods, and avoid fried food.

8. Be smoke free. Smoking lowers the HDL (good) cholesterol in the blood.
9. Get physically active most days of the week. Being active *raises* your HDL.
10. If you are overweight, losing pounds can help normalize your cholesterol levels. I'm a firm believer that weight loss should be gradual and sensible through portion control and healthier eating.

Treating high triglycerides is slightly different from treating LDL cholesterol. Your risk for heart disease is increased if you have high triglycerides. That may be because people with high triglycerides have a greater tendency for diabetes or low HDL levels. Regardless, you should make the effort to lower triglycerides through diet and lifestyle choices. Triglycerides can be controlled by reducing simple sugars in your diet, cutting down on alcohol and trying to reduce the extra weight across your waist. Some people with very high triglycerides (which we define as more than 10 mmol/L, or millimoles per litre) are at risk of inflammation of the pancreas, or pancreatitis. These are the patients who need to be on triglyceride medications. If you have heart disease and have very high triglycerides requiring medication, make sure you are on the other types of cholesterol medications (statins) as well.

Manage Your Blood Pressure

Treating hypertension is important at every age, especially in the elderly. A recent study concluded that patients over age 80 who use medications to decrease blood pressure are at lower risk of death, stroke and congestive heart failure.

If you have high blood pressure, a home monitor is useful. Blood pressure should be measured when you are relaxed and rested because people have higher readings when they are under physical or emotional stress. I recommend sitting down and measuring your BP at the same time of day for every reading. Of course, many patients tell me "they're always too stressed" when the blood pressure cuff goes on. If you are that rare individual, consider relaxation exercises, and talk to your doctor about stress management techniques.

If you are measuring your blood pressure at home, make sure you are using an approved device. A list of devices is available on the Hypertension Canada website, www.hypertension.ca. If your home blood pressure monitor does not seem to be giving you the same readings as in your doctor's office, take it in and check your blood pressure with both devices at the same time to ensure it's working correctly.

I strongly believe you should take charge of your health, without allowing a health concern to cripple you. I have many patients in my practice who are on good blood pressure medications and have adopted the right lifestyle changes. They seem to be obsessed with monitoring blood pressure several times per day. It is more important to adopt a healthier lifestyle and take your medications than to be consumed with numbers that may very well be in the normal range for you. Plus, blood pressure will normally fluctuate during the day. An occasional high reading usually is nothing to worry about.

Salt reduction, weight loss and physical activity are important interventions that affect your blood pressure. Regardless of what you may have heard about the benefits of red wine, reducing your alcohol intake is better for your blood pressure, too. If you have high blood pressure and cut your drinking from three glasses of alcohol a day to one or zero, you can lower your blood pressure by an average of 4 systolic units (or mm Hg, the top number in a BP reading) and 2.5 diastolic units (the bottom number). For example, you can go from a blood pressure of 160/90 to 156/88 just by cutting out the booze. If you are exercising for a minimum of 30 minutes at a time, three times per week, you can lower blood pressure by more than 10 systolic units (on the top) and about 7 diastolic units (on the bottom). That is, you can lower your blood pressure from 150/80 to 140/73 just by being active. That's as good as the effect of some pills that people take for hypertension.

As for diet, the concept is to decrease the amount of fat intake from meats and to eat more fruits and vegetables and foods high in potassium (except if you have kidney disease, which is not a good pairing with potassium). Tomatoes have the highest potassium content and are low in calories. Oranges and bananas are high in potassium too but are also higher in calories.

I seldom recommend specific diets, save to say that the DASH diet is pretty good and medically validated for hypertension. DASH stands for Dietary Approaches to Stop Hypertension, and the diet is supported by the American-based National Heart Lung and Blood Institute. It's a plan for eating to keep blood pressure in check, and it emphasizes a diet rich in potassium, magnesium and calcium—all of which are associated with lower blood pressure. The DASH diet includes fresh fruits and vegetables plus low-fat or non-fat dairy. On this diet, you keep sodium intake low and concentrate on eating more servings of fresh produce and whole grains a day, while keeping a tight control on consuming low amounts of red meats, fats and sweets. The DASH diet is also rich in fish, poultry, legumes and seeds.[11]

The diet can lower blood pressure by more than 10 units (systolic) and 5 units (diastolic). Your risk for heart attack and stroke will be lower too!

That said, I don't tell my patients to get on the DASH diet first off, since I truly believe that lifestyle choices and moderation in dietary intake are best for most of us. But if you are having difficulty controlling your blood pressure, then the DASH diet is a reasonable plan.

Many of you with heart disease may need medications for blood pressure control—perhaps up to three or four types of pills. The good news is that many blood pressure pills are effective. Which one is the best is a matter of tremendous debate and the topic of constant studies, each with a seemingly different conclusion. At the end of the day, I say it doesn't really matter what medication you are on, as long as it's controlling your blood pressure. It's simple: Stay on your medications as prescribed, check your blood pressure at home (or in the drugstore) and discuss the results with your doctor.

♥ **You need to know: Stay on your medications as prescribed, check your blood pressure at home (or in the drugstore) and discuss the results with your doctor. The type of blood pressure medication usually doesn't matter if you are otherwise healthy. All blood pressure medications are more useful when you are eating well, exercising regularly and trying to maintain a healthy body weight.**

You may, like many people, not wish to take medications for the rest of your life. That's one of the big issues with blood pressure control. Many of you may not be entirely convinced that drugs designed to prevent illness are working, because you never *see* the stroke or heart attack you are preventing. The daily benefits of medication are virtually invisible to us unless we go in to the doctor for a medical test.

Research shows that within one year, up to 50% of patients will discontinue their prescription drugs, including cholesterol and blood pressure meds.[12] An additional 35% of people will discontinue treatment within two years. Many are fearful of side effects or don't "see" the benefit of the drug in a way that is tangible to them. But the flip side is that most people don't experience serious side effects while on medications that are beneficial to them. Ultimately, the greater benefit is leading a longer, healthier life, free from heart attack and stroke.

I can't stress enough that preventing heart disease and stroke is the goal—and medications play a big part in saving lives. Think of blood pressure pills as "stroke prevention pills." I also advise family members of patients to check in and make sure their loved ones continue to take their medications. Simple

If you're in your 80s and are on hypertension medication, you might be wondering about the risk versus reward of taking the drugs. In the past, physicians have debated whether lowering blood pressure in very elderly people could cause more harm than good. Although the higher your blood pressure, the higher your risk of stroke, some population studies suggest that patients age 80 or older had better survival rates with higher levels of blood pressure. This was countered by the international HYVET study, which stands for Hypertension in the Very Elderly Trial. This large trial found that most subjects—averaging 83.5 years of age with an average blood pressure of 173/90—saw a significant reduction in strokes and congestive heart failure and death while on blood pressure medication.[13]

pill boxes are useful. Many patients have blister packs—medications dispensed by the pharmacist that need to be opened every day according to a schedule. Keep your medications in an area where you will see them as part of a routine—near your toothbrush or your coffee pot, for instance.

Control Your Diabetes

As mentioned in Chapter 2, Type 2 diabetes (or adult-onset diabetes) is related to the inability to process or handle the insulin that the pancreas makes. Insulin is the hormone that helps you lower the level of glucose in your blood; glucose is the sugar that gets broken down from the food we eat. Diabetes has a strong link to cardiovascular disease. In type 2 diabetes, glucose and insulin levels are higher than normal. These abnormal values can lead to atherosclerosis—the disease where plaque builds up in your arteries.

Many of the effects of type 2 diabetes can be managed by maintaining the many principles of prevention we've covered in this chapter. Focusing on diet and exercise may not only reduce your requirements for diabetes medications but also will have a positive impact on cardiovascular health. You can help manage your diabetes and improve your heart health by eating balanced, healthy meals and following a plan for physical activity. You can develop diabetes if you are overweight, so it's important to maintain a healthy weight. In addition, don't smoke, keep your blood pressure and cholesterol levels low, and take your medication. Monitor your blood glucose levels if you have diabetes.

As with any element of prevention, it's important to be informed and seek a medical expert to guide you through dealing with diabetes. I see patients daily who have been diagnosed with diabetes but have never had a good dose of diabetic education. Talk to your doctor about sending you to a diabetes teaching session with a nurse educator or dietitian. These programs are invaluable.

We've now covered the basics of prevention for heart health. This chapter might have seemed like reading a guide to virtuous living in a perfect world. But of course, nobody *is* perfect. You cannot expect to turn off bad habits accumulated over a lifetime as quickly as a flip of a switch. To achieve long-lasting results, you have to develop a sustainable plan for healthy living. My best advice to you is this: Don't do it alone. Gather information from your doctors and a cheering section consisting of your friends and loved ones. The last thing you need to feel is that you're isolated in your quest. You can't have your family enjoying a big, rich, indulgent meal as a means of "celebrating," while you are on your own with a plate of steamed kale. Just as you don't want to be too hard on yourself and too impatient to reach tangible results, you also don't want to be unsupported in your quest to lose weight. Enlist a friend, spouse or relative to travel the path with you, and don't make food the centre of celebrations. Instead, go for a manicure, buy yourself a shirt you've been eyeing, play a round of golf or give yourself extra time to read a good book. There are many ways to celebrate a job well done.

5

SYMPTOMS

"I'm having chest pains and I'm not sure what to make of them. What exactly does angina feel like? Is it serious?"

Let me put you in the shoes of two people, each in a different scenario. Tell me which one you believe is related to heart disease.

In scenario number 1, you are a 67-year-old man. It is the middle of the afternoon. You have been fighting a feeling of fatigue on and off all day. In the last hour, as you've walked the dog around the block, you've had to rest to catch your breath an unusual number of times. It's not like you to be so weary, but then again you are not the young man you used to be. Six months ago, you retired from your career as a lawyer, and ever since then, you have been indulging in celebratory dinners and drinks (a few too many steaks and cigars, at times). You're staving off some of the boredom that comes with retirement by filling up your time with restaurant lunches with old colleagues as well as dinners out with your family and friends. You like to order comfort food—and you've enjoyed every gargantuan portion that has come your way. You have gained 12 pounds in half a year! At least you're still walking the dog—once in a while. But today it isn't going that well. You finally make your way around the neighbourhood and to the end of your driveway. It takes a big push of exertion to get inside. As you find your way to the sofa, you realize that a sense of heaviness in your chest hasn't left you. It's like nothing you've experienced before—a very heavy feeling of someone almost pressing down on your chest. You are tired and you can't catch your breath. After a little while, the heaviness starts to dull, only to be replaced by a realization that you've been feeling queasy too. You pick up the phone and dial 9-1-1 or your local emergency number.

In scenario number 2, you are a 49-year-old woman. Today is Saturday, which means you can take it easy—relatively speaking. You don't have to take your turn in the carpool, pack the lunches and complete the pre-dawn meal prep of that day's dinner for the kids. That was yesterday. Now, it is a day of rest. It's 7:45 in the morning. The sensation you felt on and off all day the day before—kind of like terrible indigestion—has come back. You're not sure that indigestion comes with a tightness across your entire chest and down your left arm, but that's what you feel. When you woke up at dawn, you were feeling tired and generally not yourself. You dressed, folded one pile of laundry and popped in a fresh load, and did 10 minutes on the treadmill in the basement before you could no longer go on because your symptoms were getting worse. You took an antacid to see if the discomfort would go away. A strange wave is coming over you, like carsickness, and you also start to feel hot and sweaty. You try to put it out of your mind because your kids need you to take them to their karate class. Maybe it's the flu; maybe it's something you ate. You feel awful as the discomfort radiates in your arm and up your jaw. Did you read somewhere that pain in your arm might be a heart attack? Your breathing is difficult, and you can't seem to catch enough air. You pick up the phone, and after a few moments of trying to steady yourself, you dial your sister to see what she knows about heart attacks. After all, she was around when your father had a heart attack 20 years ago.

So which of these people has a potentially life-threatening problem, the man or the woman? Of course, it's both of them. Each of these people responded differently to their experience with a chest pain we call angina. It didn't take long for the first subject to call 9-1-1—bravo. But the younger woman ignored feeling unwell, even after more than a day. She was not connecting her symptoms to what they could be related to: the fact that her heart was not getting enough blood.

Coronary heart disease has a variety of symptoms. On the following pages, you'll find detailed descriptions of the kind people commonly experience—beginning with one of the most defining symptoms, chest pain. Keep in mind as you read this primer that this chapter is not meant to *replace* a discussion with your health care professional. If you or a loved one is having chest pain, it's essential to have the specific case evaluated by a qualified physician. If you have chest pain and you believe it may be heart related, always seek emergency medical care.

Common Causes of Chest Pain

Your heart is situated slightly to the left of your breastbone, midway up your chest. But it's important to know that not all pain in the chest area comes from the heart. Conversely, not all pain that is related to the heart is felt in the chest. Cardiologists are most concerned when the cause of your pain is a lack of blood flow to your heart. This is usually a consequence of atherosclerosis (junk in the arteries). The medical term for this chest pain is *angina.* When angina lasts more than 20 minutes at a time, you are at risk of causing heart-muscle damage and having a heart attack.

When your heart cries out for blood, if you're lucky, you will have symptoms—like chest pain or difficulty breathing. Seek medical help without delay. In some situations—traditionally, if you have diabetes—you may not be fortunate enough to experience any warning symptoms. Patients with diabetes may lose sensitivity in their nerves, including those that signal pain from the heart.

❤ **You need to know: Chest pain coming from lack of blood flow to the heart is a blaring siren. Angina is a warning sign. If it lasts more than 20 minutes, you are at risk of having a heart attack. Call for an ambulance.**

Chest pain has many causes. It can be related to the heart, lungs or musculoskeletal system; to stress or anxiety; and even to the gastrointestinal tract. That last one may surprise you. In fact, the nerve supply to the heart is the same as the nerve supply to the stomach—though this is a bit of a simplification. Much of my day is taken up by figuring out if a patient's pain is coming from the heart or from a GI issue, such as an ulcer or gastroesophageal reflux disease (GERD). Only a doctor can "tease out" the root cause of chest pains. Always err on the side of caution, and discuss your pain with your physician. Rush to the emergency room if the tightness or heaviness in the chest lasts for more than 20 minutes at a time.

❤ **You need to know: Chest pain can be caused by a variety of factors, including heart, lung, stomach, muscular or stress-related problems. Only a doctor can determine the true source of the pain.**

So how can you tell if you have angina? As a rule, chest pain due to the heart often comes on with activity and goes away with rest—that is, it's *exertional.* If you have a narrowing of blood flow in your coronary arteries, your heart is usually able to compensate for the restricted flow, to some degree, when it is resting. Your arteries are complex organs. If one is narrowed, then another artery downstream from the narrowing will try to dilate (open up). But it can dilate only so much on its own. Doctors use angina medication such as nitroglycerine (which comes in a spray or pills) to dilate the blood vessels and improve blood flow to the heart to reduce angina symptoms.

If you have a narrowing in blood flow to the heart when you're active—whether it's running, walking, gardening or chasing after children—the increased demands on your heart may not be met. The same applies when you're under emotional stress. If you can walk through your chest pain, or your pain goes away the longer you remain active, it's less likely to be coming from your heart. Also, if you are at rest and having chest pains, it's not usually due to coronary heart disease—unless you're having a heart attack.

❤ **You need to know: Chest pain due to the heart often comes on with activity and goes away with rest—that is, it's *exertional.***

We've all seen a movie where a person has a heart attack, and he'll suddenly clutch the top of his arm. In fact, chest pain coming from the heart can radiate not only into arms but also to the neck, jaw, back and shoulder blades. It seldom, if ever, goes above the nose or below the belly button. I've had many people come into my office complaining of exertional headache, leg pain and lower back ache—these are not cardiac issues.

When Chest Pain Is Serious

According to the Heart and Stroke Foundation, warning signs of a heart attack include shortness of breath and/or sudden discomfort that does not go away. Remember that the pain may be in your chest, neck, jaw, shoulder, arm or back. These require urgent medical attention. If the pain occurs during activity and does *not* occur at rest, then it is usually safe to make a doctor's appointment for the following day rather than rush to the emergency room. In any event, make sure you see a doctor, and empower yourself by making a point-blank inquiry: "Could this be my heart?" Asking the right questions will help protect you and close any gaps in your care.

♥ You need to know: You need to call 9-1-1 or your local emergency number if

- **your chest pain does not go away with rest or lasts for more than 20 minutes at a time. After 20 minutes of lack of blood flow to your heart, you may be at risk of heart muscle damage.**
- **your chest pain is radiating into the arms, neck, jaw, back and shoulder blades. The pain usually does not go above your nose or below your belly button.**
- **you feel severe shortness of breath, nausea or indigestion; you are vomiting, sweating or feeling cool or clammy; or you have a sudden sensation of severe light headedness.**

Heart-related pain may feel like burning, squeezing, heaviness, tightness or pressure. Discomfort that's brought on with exertion and goes away with rest can be a sign that a heart attack is impending. (Whereas if you're actually having an attack, the discomfort will simply not go away.) Other symptoms include shortness of breath, difficulty breathing, nausea, indigestion, vomiting, sweating or feeling cool and clammy, or a sudden onset of severe light-headedness. If you are experiencing any of these signs, call 9-1-1 immediately.

Asking the right questions can be life-saving. My mother, Dolores, is living proof. Although my mother is a teacher, we joke that she's the third cardiologist in the family—she's been happily married to one for 45 years. Several years ago, her friend, a woman in her 60s, experienced pain in her shoulder. She reported it to her family doctor, who worked her up with X-rays to see if it was arthritis. The unusual aspect of this pain was that it occurred only when my mother's friend rushed around taking care of her grandchildren. She got relief when she rested. My mom knew this sounded like a coronary issue, so she strongly suggested that her friend revisit her symptoms with her physician. The doctor ultimately performed a stress test and made a diagnosis of coronary heart disease. In fact, Mom's friend went on to have bypass surgery and, I'm happy to say, 10 years later, she's doing well.

Angina and heart attack occur more commonly in someone at risk. Therefore, if you are middle-aged or older, and if you smoke or have diabetes, high blood pressure or high cholesterol, then in general the chest pain may be more serious than it is for younger, healthier individuals without these risk factors. Discuss your symptoms with your physician.

For a doctor, a "Hollywood heart attack"—that is, a classic one you might see in a movie—is when you describe "an elephant sitting on your chest." People who arrive in the ER with a heart attack often have a sudden onset of chest discomfort that feels new and unusual. It may not be the full elephant. Often, there's a squeezing sensation, and the patient will have difficulty breathing, will have a grey appearance, and will feel cold or clammy or suddenly light-headed.

Blood tests will determine if the heart muscle has developed microscopic damage because of lack of blood flow. Sometimes, chest pain is due to a rupture or tear in the aorta, which presents as excruciating chest or back pain. Aortic tears are more often seen in older people who have high blood pressure.

❤ **You need to know: If you or your family member has a new symptom of chest, arm, throat or jaw discomfort, or a shortness of breath that comes on with activity and goes away with rest, then talk to your doctor sooner rather than later.**

Non-Serious Chest Pain

Your doctor can determine if your chest pain is heart related by assessing your symptoms. Pinpoint, needle-like or sharp stabbing pains, usually smaller than a quarter, are not cardiac problems. However, if you feel a pressure-like discomfort or heaviness in the chest, often described as a "vice-like pain," this may be due to heart disease. With a heart attack, many of you will describe symptoms as heavy discomfort rather than pain. The discomfort can often be severe enough to restrict movement. Rarely will it be sharp in nature and cause you to writhe. Irritation or sharp pain can be caused by an inflammation of the sac surrounding the heart (pericarditis)—but this is less common. Pain that is worse if you take a deep breath doesn't usually come from the heart; it is likelier to come from a problem related to the lungs. Often doctors describe pain that changes with breathing as pleuritic pain, meaning lung related, for which there are serious and non-serious causes. You should get this sorted by seeing a doctor.

"Silent" Heart Problems

So-called silent heart attacks are heart attacks that don't come with chest pain. They usually occur in people who are at risk of heart disease—particularly women over 60, men over 50 or anyone with a heart risk factor. (For a full breakdown of the risks, see Chapter 2.)

But these heart attacks are really not "silent." If you suddenly feel severely unwell, nauseous or weak, it's possibly the result of problems with the heart. Obviously not everyone who feels unwell is having a heart attack—more likely, the culprit will be something more common, such as the flu. It's best to see your doctor within a few days and ask if your symptoms could be your heart.

Shortness of Breath

The medical term for shortness of breath is *dyspnea*, derived from the Latin words for abnormal (*dys*) and breath (*pnea*). Sometimes being short of breath with exertion is just a sign that you are out of shape. Other causes can be lung related, anything as common as a simple upper respiratory tract infection or as serious as pneumonia. If your blood levels are low, or you're anemic, you may also be short of breath.

❤ **You need to know: Common causes of shortness of breath include heart disease, lung problems and just being out of shape.**

Shortness of breath that's exertional could be your heart. When you are short of breath on exertion but do *not* have chest discomfort, doctors worry this may be an angina equivalent. This means the symptoms are coming from blood-flow issues, even if they don't show up as chest pains. At first glance, it's tough for your doctor to know what exactly is going on if you are short of breath. You can have these symptoms just because you are out of shape. The catch is, if you are out of shape, you may also have risk factors for heart disease such as obesity, diabetes or high blood pressure. Ultimately, your physician may need to do a stress test (see Chapter 6) or a lung function test.

Some clues to coronary heart disease are fairly obvious. For instance, I have a 55-year-old patient who was part of a running group. Normally, she could readily keep up with her jogging buddies. But she suddenly found herself falling behind. I ordered a stress test because her symptoms could not be explained by being out of shape. We discovered that she had a narrowing of her left anterior descending artery (LAD; see Chapter 1), which was causing her to slow down and be out of breath. In contrast, another patient of mine had high blood pressure and gained 30 pounds in four years. The weight gain had come as a result of her stress. She was dealing with a difficult situation with elder care and did not feel she had the time to make her health a priority. She was not short of breath in ordinary instances of activity. This woman's case was very different from the jogger, who found that she suddenly couldn't keep up a regular routine. In the latter, the woman had to lose weight and adopt a habit of regular exercise and see her family doctor after six months. After a while, her symptoms were resolved.

❤ **You need to know: If you're generally fit but, out of the blue, you find it hard to keep up with regular activities because you are winded, then talk to your doctor. It might be your heart. On the other hand, if, as part of your New Year's resolution, you went back to the gym for the first time in years trying to shed gained weight, then it's normal to feel shortness of breath, because your body is out of shape. Take it slowly at first. Consult your doctor if the shortness of breath doesn't resolve itself the fitter you become.**

When your heart doesn't pump efficiently, pressures can build up in the left side of the heart and in your lungs. High pressures in the lungs, or pulmonary hypertension, may cause shortness of breath. Pulmonary hypertension is serious and may be caused by a heart-muscle or valve-related problem. In rare cases, it's due to a very serious lung disease. Your doctor can sort out the cause with a chest X-ray, ultrasound of the heart (or echocardiogram) and lung (pulmonary) function tests.

Shortness of breath due to congestive heart failure—when the pump itself isn't working—is positional. That means it's usually worse when you lie down and better when you sit up. These breathing problems can creep up in the middle of the night. With heart failure, you may wake up gasping for air—a result of fluid building up in your lungs when you sleep. Patients with congestive heart failure also may experience coughing due to fluid in the lungs. In contrast, patients with coronary blood flow problems—a different and serious condition—may sometimes have shortness of breath only on exertion. In these patients, as well as those with lung disease, breathing issues aren't positional. We cover heart failure in depth in Chapter 12.

Feeling Weak, Light-Headed or Dizzy

You may visit your doctor complaining that you feel weak, light-headed and dizzy. Let's take it one piece at a time and start with your symptoms of weakness. In general, if you have a normal-functioning heart muscle—that is, the pump is squeezing well—then your weakness is not usually related to the heart.

Light-headedness is a different story. Feeling light-headed, or as if you're about to faint, could be a sign that your heart is not pumping efficiently. Light-headedness is not the same as experiencing a dizzy sensation—or spinning. In general, if the room is spinning (vertigo), it's more likely due to an inner-ear problem.

Sometimes, light-headedness may also be related to the effects of heart or blood pressure medication; your pills may be too powerful and lower the blood pressure too much. It's rare to feel light-headed if your systolic blood pressure (the top number) is more than 110. In fact, many times I've heard patients say, "My blood pressure is too low and I'm light-headed," but when I check the BP, it's 120/70, which is entirely normal.

Another common cause of light-headedness is orthostatic hypotension, which means your blood pressure falls sharply when you quickly stand up. You may experience orthostatic hypotension if you are older and your blood vessels are not at optimal health, or if you take multiple blood pressure medications. Doctors can diagnose it by checking blood pressure twice—when you are lying down and then while standing—to see if there's a significant fall in between. Treating orthostatic hypotension is often simple: Your doctor may advise you to sit up slowly and not to rush. Support stockings are also a great help because they prevent the blood from pooling in the legs. In my experience, however, patients don't wear support hose as much as they should—vanity!

❤ **You need to know: With orthostatic hypotension, your blood pressure falls when you stand up quickly from a seated or lying position. This is usually seen in older people. Often the treatment is to take it easy getting up or to wear support hose to keep blood from pooling in the legs.**

Fainting

It may seem like one of the more dramatic things to ever happen to your body—you hear a ringing in your ears, the voices around you get more distant, perhaps you feel nauseous, and suddenly you open your eyes to discover you've fallen. Fainting can be alarming. Also known by the medical term *syncope*, fainting results from a temporary lack of oxygen to the brain. But it can be caused by simple reasons. When it comes to your heart, if you are an otherwise young, healthy person, fainting is not usually a cause for concern. But it's a major cause of concern if you have a fast heart rate and you've already had a heart attack in the past. I'll explain.

There's non-serious fainting, called a vasovagal episode. If you get sick at the sight of blood or are under emotional stress, you may experience a "simple faint," usually seen in otherwise healthy individuals who have low normal blood pressures. Believe it or not, this kind of fainting is a sign that your nervous system is healthy. The autonomic nervous system of your body is a finely tuned machine. Under normal circumstances, if someone yells "boo" and you jump out of your skin, your nervous system will release adrenalin, your heart will race and your blood pressure will rise. Adrenalin release can also happen because of a stress on the body or when you are in pain or ill. To ensure that your blood pressure doesn't rise to the point of a stroke or heart attack, the autonomic nervous system stimulates a nerve that counterbalances the effect of adrenalin. This is the vagus nerve. Think of it as a stop-sign nerve because when stimulated, it dilates your vessels to lower your blood pressure and slow down your heart rate. A "simple faint" is called a vasovagal attack.

If you're very healthy and fit, your stop sign tends to be activated more often, even at rest. This means you have a lower heart rate and lower normal blood pressure than most people. Olympic athletes often have low resting heart rates because their nervous systems are "turned on"—their bodies have learned to deal with increased adrenalin by ramping up the stop-sign nerve. Some healthy young people may have an overactive vagus nerve as well. When they're scared or under stress, to counterbalance the release of adrenalin, the vagus nerve fires away at an increased rate, telling the heart rate to slow down and causing their blood pressure to fall. When this occurs, they might feel light-headed or faint.

Usually, you have a warning sign that you're about to faint because the vagus nerve takes time to lower the blood pressure. You may hear ringing in your ears. You might also be nauseous or feel the sudden urge to go to the bathroom.

Simple faints triggered by your fight-or-flight response may have been necessary in caveman times, but today, none of us really needs an overactive stop-sign nerve. Still, many people experience fainting. If you're a repeat fainter, you should try to avoid triggers—avoid the horror movie, for example, and see a romantic comedy. Make sure that under times of stress, your body temperature is not overheated (which often makes the effects of the vagus nerve worse). Keep up with drinking fluids and eating food because the vagus nerve is more likely to activate when you are running on empty. Eat your breakfast in the morning, and let yourself (in this case only) have a little more salt intake than usual as you load up with fluids. Eating a low-fat snack such as salted pretzels or drinking fluids containing salt, such as Gatorade and V8 juice, may solve simple fainting.

❤ **You need to know: If you are a fainter, you should increase your intake of salt, food and fluids when you are under stress. Avoid alcohol in stressful situations.**

I've been a fainter since I was nine. The first time it happened, I was in Girl Guides. When I fainted, an adult called an ambulance. Unfortunately, the person who phoned my mom panicked and told her she thought I might be dead. In the last 10 years, I've fainted a handful of times when there's been extreme stress on my body, like when I had a knee injury when skiing. (In situations like this I will ask a medical colleague of mine, who happens to be the national authority on fainting, to email my mother and assure her I'm okay). I know that certain scenarios, like being cramped on an airplane, are fainting triggers. When you're squished on a plane, blood can pool in the legs. That's why it's a good idea to drink only water and non-alcoholic drinks when flying. (Alcohol is bad for fainters because it is a vasodilator and opens up your blood vessels). And if you do feel that ringing sensation or nausea, get into a position where you have more blood going to your brain. Sit down and put your head to your knees so your head is below your heart. Or lie down on the floor and put your feet up.

Then there's serious fainting. In these cases, you lose consciousness without warning. Serious faints are often severe enough to cause bruising, bleeding or other injuries. Often, they are the result of irregular heartbeats, or arrhythmias—the rhythm problems of the heart. If you are older, your heart may beat too slowly and may cause you to faint. Or you may faint because of a fast heart rate (tachycardia). This is especially a cause for concern if you've had a previous heart attack and your heart muscle has been damaged. (A heart attack can lead to a short-circuit in your heart and to arrhythmia.) Usually the treatment for a fast heart rate, in addition to medication, is an implantable defibrillator or a procedure called an ablation (described in Chapter 11). That said, remember that if a fast heartbeat causes you to faint but your heart is otherwise normal, your situation likely isn't serious in the big picture. Talk to your doctor to sort out if your fainting symptoms are serious.

In rare situations, you may have a special pacemaker implanted in your body to treat extreme simple fainting. The pacemaker will have special qualities that ramp up the heart rate (the medical term is *hysteresis*) around the time of a faint. But this doesn't always work. I recall quite vividly being a cardiology resident and being called to a code blue, meaning the patient had no detectable pulse. The patient had just come back from a pacemaker insertion for a simple faint. The pacemaker had worked, but it did not resolve her low blood pressure or keep her blood vessels from dilating, which had caused her to pass out. Fortunately, this patient came to.

In addition, if you have aortic valve problems, you might be susceptible to a serious faint because the calcium that builds up in the aortic valve could extend into the electrical system, causing the heart to "block" or slow down (see Chapter 11).

You can also lose consciousness from fainting if you have circulatory problems or seizure disorders. A clue that a seizure is causing the problem is when there's arm or leg movement, mouth biting, frothing or loss of bowel or bladder functions during a loss of consciousness. This needs to be taken seriously.

Palpitations

Palpitations are quite common. People who experience them describe the symptoms in a variety of ways. Often you may feel a sensation of "thumping" or extra heartbeats. You might say your heart is racing or "flying out of your chest." All of these are palpitations. But interestingly, palpitations are not always caused by heart disease. Of every 10 patients I see in my office for palpitations, five have a true rhythm problem of the heart (such as arrhythmia) and five do not.

If you are having palpitations related to stress and anxiety, chances are you're not imagining things. Stress-related palpitations mean that subconsciously your brain is playing tricks on your body. The extreme example of this is a panic attack, when you feel you can't breathe, your heart is racing and you have a sense of impending doom. Your doctor can determine if stress, anxiety or true arrhythmia is to blame for your palpitations by having you wear a heart-monitoring device called a Holter (see Chapter 7). If stress and anxiety are the cause, you may benefit from talking through your issues with people you trust or engaging in regular relaxation exercises such as yoga or deep breathing.

❤ **You need to know:** **If you are under excess stress, you may have palpitations that are not due to a heart problem. Deep breathing techniques can help: Breathe in for three seconds, hold for three seconds, and slowly breathe out for three seconds several times throughout the day to deal with the symptoms and bring the stress levels back to baseline.**

If you describe having a chest pain at the same time as experiencing palpitations, that may be a clue that your palpitations are not serious. An irregular heartbeat does not usually go hand in hand with chest pain. Some people may experience a sensation of palpitations due to extra heartbeats, whether they're at the top part of the heart (called supraventricular beats) or the bottom part of the heart (ventricular beats). We go into detail on the nature of extra beats in Chapter 9. They are usually not serious if you are otherwise healthy, do not have heart-muscle damage and are not fainting.

Cramps, Aches and Fatigue in the Legs

If you have disease in your leg arteries, you will commonly have circulation problems and difficulty walking. This is called claudication—cramps, aches, soreness or fatigue in the legs, usually in the calf muscles, that comes on with activity and goes away with rest. Claudication is angina of the legs, a symptom of serious circulation problems and peripheral arterial disease. Your doctor can give you a simple, non-invasive test to assess claudication (see Chapter 7).

❤ **You need to know:** **If you have cramping in your calves every time you walk—and it goes away with rest—you need to talk to your doctor to test for a circulation problem.**

Do Women's Symptoms Differ from Men's?

For some reason that is unclear to me, the media have perpetuated a myth that women may have different symptoms than men. (We tackle this topic in depth in Chapter 3.) This is the sexy topic du jour people want to discuss when I talk about women and heart disease. But it's not at all true. With a heart attack, men feel heaviness in their chests, shortness of breath, nausea or other general discomfort—but so, too, can women.[1] One true difference is that many women communicate differently than men, or they will minimize the gravity of their condition because they simply have a lot on the go. They can't imagine how on earth their families or their bosses can survive without them. In so many ways, women are classic type E personalities: Everything to everyone except themselves. This mentality may cause women to soldier on in the face of pain or crisis, perilously risking their health in the process.

As a matter of course in my life, I always try to remind people how crucial it is to ask for help. There's no such thing as stoic nobility. When I hear that patients suffered through chest pains and other warning signs, I'm unequivocal: Doing nothing is not a good course of action. One of the most important things that anyone, woman or man, has to remember is that it's imperative *not* to avoid seeking medical expertise—especially when you need it most.

Next up: We examine some of the tests you may undergo when you do take the right steps and turn to medical professionals for help. These tools are essential for making a cardiac diagnosis.

PART III

Navigating the System When Something Goes Wrong

6

TESTING AND EVALUATING CHEST PAIN

"How will the doctors know if my chest pain is coming from my heart?"

We've covered the gamut of risk factors and how to protect yourself and your loved ones from developing coronary heart disease. We've reviewed the common symptoms of the disease, such as chest pain and shortness of breath, and their potential severity. Now it's time to examine the screening methods that doctors rely on to evaluate your symptoms. Physicians may conduct a range of tests in order to sort out a diagnosis and determine your treatments (see Chapters 10 through 12).

Every one of you has likely had at least some form of medical test in your life, whether it's a routine blood screen or a test involving electrodes connected to a computer. An example of the latter is an essential test in cardiac care called an electrocardiogram (or ECG, which we talk about in detail soon). But many of you are unaware of the exact purpose and value of these tests. Especially in an emergency situation, you may receive only a cursory explanation of why blood is being drawn from your arm or why leads are being stuck to your chest.

Some tests are conducted by your cardiologist or family doctor in his practice; others are given in a hospital ER. The pages that follow provide a base of knowledge on the types of evaluations for heart disease. We'll cover the principles of the key tests, where and why they are given, how they work and what level of information they provide for your doctors. Understanding these screenings and the contexts in which they're used will help you prepare for any tests that lie ahead. You want to know about these tests for the same reasons you need to know about your risks and symptoms: to feel secure about asking the right questions of the right medical professionals at the right times.

Any testing comes hand in hand with a dialogue. Whether you're seeing a cardiologist or your family doctor or you find yourself at a hospital window marked *triage,* you will be asked a series of important questions. Doctors will want to know the relevant details about your symptoms, such as when you experience them, their duration and your medical history. Don't feel anxious about remembering every detail to the minute. None of us has the ability to recall the minutiae. Do your best, but remember that questions are just one part of evaluation. The medical tests will tell your doctors what's actually going on in your body. Here's a thorough rundown of the six main tests we use when you have chest pain and what you should expect from them.

Electrocardiogram

An electrocardiogram is otherwise known as an ECG, an EKG or simply a cardiogram. It's the main initial test that doctors use to diagnose cardiac problems. It's a measurement of the electrical activity of your heart, and it's obtained by putting electrodes, or leads, on your chest, arms and legs. Usually the ECG reading is displayed on a piece of paper; sometimes it's shown on a monitor.

A traditional ECG looks at the heart in different aspects, providing 12 specific views of electrical activity. The test takes less than five minutes and does not require any special preparation. You just need to lie flat for the recording.

The ECG detects the rhythm of the heart, whether it's normal or irregular. The test will show if you've had a substantial heart attack, because in the area where the heart muscle has died, there will be no electrical activity. The ECG will also measure a temporary lack of blood flow to your heart (known as ischemia) provided the test is performed when you are experiencing pain. If an ECG is performed when your pain is gone, the results may be normal. However, if the cause of your pain is a serious and prolonged lack of blood flow to the heart, the ECG will often (but not always) register minor abnormalities in electrical activity. The ECG may also give cardiologists clues to a thickening heart muscle, or enlargement in your heart chambers. Your doctor will use other tests, such as an echocardiogram (see Chapter 7), to confirm if your heart is enlarged.

In women, as in men, the heart is underneath the breast tissue. However, a woman's breasts have more tissue than a man's. This is why in women, when doctors measure the electrical impulses with an ECG, or we take pictures (or scans) to assess the activity of the heart, the breast tissue sometimes gets in the way. This may blur the pictures and give us falsely abnormal results. Talk to your doctor about the chances of this happening and what you and your physician can do to ensure that test results are accurate.

An ECG can be performed in a cardiologist's practice, in your family doctor's office or in an emergency room. It's usually one of the first tests you'll receive if you're rushed to an ER for angina or if you are in the midst of a heart attack. If you have the test while your heart attack is in progress, the ECG can detect a serious abnormality in electrical activity caused by lack of blood flow to the heart. This lets your doctor know to either prescribe clot-busting medication (see Chapter 10) or take you straight to a catheterization lab in order to open up the narrowed artery with an angioplasty (see Chapter 10).

That said, the ECG won't do everything. It will not directly tell you the status of any narrowings in your vessels. That's because your heart is smart enough to compensate for its lack of blood flow. If the flow in an artery is restricted, the part of the artery downstream from the blockage can open up to accommodate the movement of blood. It's like driving on a highway during roadwork. If the highway has an extra lane open, you're less likely to be slowed down by the construction.

The ECG will also not give you specific information about the state of your heart valves or heart-muscle problems, nor will it help assess your future risk for heart disease. In other words, you can have a normal ECG but still be at significantly increased risk—for example, if you're a person with high blood pressure or diabetes.

If you have chest pain, an ECG is a necessary test. As a cardiologist, I almost always order an ECG when I do a physical exam. I rely on the information the ECG and other heart tests provide to make a diagnosis.

Abnormal results from an ECG may cause you great concern. Patients often walk into my office holding their ECGs, very worried about the findings on the computer printout. But there's where a cardiologist comes in! The fact is, often a computer analysis will "overcall" abnormalities that doctors consider nonspecific. Meaning certain abnormalities may not, in fact, be due to any serious causes. If you or a family member is concerned about an abnormal outcome in a test, rest assured there might be nothing to worry about. Your doctor will sort it out by evaluating your results in the full context of your medical history.

Blood Tests

If you have prolonged chest discomfort or long-lasting shortness of breath, hopefully you will rush to an emergency room. There, your doctors will order blood tests to measure enzymes and biomarkers. These blood tests are a measure of heart-muscle damage. They help physicians find out if your symptoms are due to coronary heart disease—for instance, a heart attack.

Blood tests are more commonly done in an emergency room. That's because when you have a heart attack and your heart muscle is damaged, it releases a substance in the blood. The substance usually peaks within hours of the onset of symptoms and then goes away. So it's important to take blood fairly quickly, when you are in the midst of experiencing or have just had an episode of long-lasting chest pain.

Chest pain is usually a cry for help—the heart is telling you it's not receiving enough blood. After 20 to 30 minutes of lack of blood flow, your heart muscle may be damaged, either at a microscopic or substantial level. If even one or two heart-muscle cells (myocytes) are damaged, then those cells leak a chemical (enzyme) into the blood that we can detect with blood tests. The enzymes indicate if you're having a heart attack.

It may take several hours after an episode of chest pain for the heart muscle to be damaged. So doctors will often repeat the blood tests six to eight hours after the first test. They may even require a third set of enzymes before they can send you home from the ER.

There's a catch with blood tests. If you have chest discomfort that lasts only 5 to 10 minutes, the blood results may be normal. This may mean it was unlikely the chest pain was a heart attack. But your chest pain may still be related to your heart. Your doctor will need to investigate further. If your enzymes *and* your ECG come back as normal, it's usually safe for the emergency room doctor to send you home and have you be evaluated as an outpatient. If your enzymes are negative after 30 minutes of prolonged chest pain, that's good news. It's unlikely that the pain is coming from your heart.

The more abnormal the enzymes, the higher your risk for significant heart problems in the near future. In general, if you have an abnormal blood test, your doctor needs to take pictures of your heart in order to investigate further, whether that's done by a nuclear perfusion scan (see page 133) or a coronary angiogram (see page 135).

Back in the old days, doctors used a blood test called CK (creatine kinase)—a muscle enzyme used to detect muscle damage in your heart. However, the CK test is not particularly sensitive or specific to the heart. You can have an elevation in CKs for a variety of reasons that have nothing to do with the heart, such as vigorous activity or falling on the sidewalk. Some emergency departments may still be using the CK test. But a more common alternative is the troponin test, a very sensitive and specific blood test for your heart. If your doctor has detected elevated levels of a substance called troponin in your blood, you may have had damage to your heart muscle. The troponin test can be so perceptive, in fact, that it may even pick up microscopic damage from a brief but severe episode of chest pain. This sometimes means the test is too good. Even if your troponin enzymes come back as borderline abnormal, you may not actually have coronary heart disease or lack of blood flow to the heart. Your doctor needs to take a full history and possibly order other tests to make a proper diagnosis.

♥ **You need to know: The troponin blood test is a sensitive test in cardiac care. It's used to determine if you have any microscopic heart-muscle damage with chest pain. If, after 30 minutes of prolonged pain, the blood test comes back as normal, then the problem is less likely to be your heart.**

Stress Test

A stress test is another initial evaluation for chest pain. It assesses your heart during various stages of activity. Your doctor will order a stress test only if you're experiencing symptoms of the disease, such as chest pain and shortness of breath. At the start of the test, a technician will stick patches (electrocardiogram leads) to various points on your chest. You will then walk on a treadmill. As you walk on the treadmill, the speed and incline will increase, supervised by a physician. The more you exert yourself to keep up with the treadmill, the more oxygen your heart will need. As oxygen is carried to your heart muscles in the coronary arteries, if you have a narrowing of blood flow to your heart, the ECG may become abnormal on a stress test.

During the test, the ECG will monitor the electrical activity of your heart and your heart rate. The technician will check your blood pressure. If there's a serious blood-flow problem, which means your coronary arteries are narrowed by more than 50%, the stress test will indicate a positive, or abnormal, result once you are active. Having chest pain on the treadmill, but no changes on the ECG, is considered a negative, or normal, result. Cardiologists take into account how long you can walk on the treadmill before developing chest pain to determine the type of treatment you'll need. The longer and farther you go, the better off you are.

❤ **You need to know: There is usually no reason to have a stress test unless you're experiencing symptoms of heart disease.**

Sometimes a stress test will be abnormal even though you don't have heart disease. This is complicated to explain, but it basically comes down to the fact that no test is perfect. Your doctor will often need other measures to clarify a diagnosis.

As a cardiologist, I won't give you a stress test if your chance of having heart disease is low. There is no point in having the test unless you have symptoms—pain in your chest, throat, arm or jaw, or shortness of breath that comes on with activity and goes away with rest. Palpitations, or extra heartbeats, are generally not symptoms of coronary heart problems. These issues are more "electrical" than "plumbing"—they suggest a rhythm problem of the heart (see Chapter 11). As such, you likely won't need a stress test.

If you are unable to exercise on a treadmill for a stress test, doctors can imitate the effects of activity on your heart by infusing a drug such as dobutamine. This medication causes the heart to beat faster and squeeze harder. A dobutamine test usually gives the same information as a treadmill stress test, except it won't give your doctor a sense of your exercise tolerance.

❤ **You need to know: If your symptoms are unusual for coronary heart disease—for example, you are having palpitations—this may indicate an electrical problem of the heart and not a blood-flow problem. You usually won't need a stress test in this case. Having one could result in a false positive.**

It's possible to have a falsely abnormal stress test. It's also possible to have a falsely *normal* test—meaning the stress test comes out fine but the patient actually does have heart disease. If this sounds confusing, it is. Rest assured that good clinical judgment most often sorts the false results from the real. Most of you should start with preventive screening tools—by having a doctor assess your Framingham Risk Score (see Chapter 2) and by identifying and minimizing risk factors for heart disease, such as diabetes and hypertension. Generally, your doctor should recommend tests only if you're having symptoms. Unfortunately, there is no single magic test that we can perform on the entire population,

No Symptoms, No Stress Test! As a rule, you and your doctor should not seek out a stress test if you're *not* having symptoms that suggest heart disease. Ordering tests without just cause can lead to a waste of time, effort and resources. (Besides, I'm not sure we should adopt the mindset of the for-profit American system, where consumers are able to pay to obtain any number of evaluations and procedures—whether they're necessary or not.) It's concerning that in the Canadian corporate world, stress tests have recently become popular. These tests are now requested as a matter of routine, not by doctors but by HR managers! Many executive programs offer stress testing yearly for their clients, whether they are having symptoms or not. This is nothing short of a waste of time and resources—and, even worse, the evaluation can lead to falsely abnormal test results.

whether you are an executive or a stay-at-home mom, that will screen appropriately for coronary heart disease.

In fact, one test usually sets off a chain reaction of others. If a stress ECG test result is abnormal, the next step may be to order a scan of the heart, such as a stress echocardiogram (see the next section) or a nuclear perfusion scan (see page 133). If they come back looking fine, then we can say the stress ECG test was falsely abnormal. It's like the game Rock, Paper, Scissors. One move, such as a rock, will trump another, such as the scissors. In this particular case, the scan of the heart trumps the treadmill test.

You need a stress test only if you have symptoms or a doctor is concerned that you have heart disease. You may be a 60-year-old man who is generally healthy despite being in the age target zone for heart disease. You may have no symptoms of the disease, but if you have a treadmill test, there is a chance you may have a falsely positive result. That is, your ECG reading will change on the treadmill even though the blood flow to your heart is normal. In this case, appearances can be deceiving. Now take a vibrant 50-year-old female executive and put her on the treadmill. Statistically, a younger woman's likelihood of having heart disease is much lower than the older man's chances. The younger woman is also more likely to have a falsely positive, or falsely abnormal, test result. This logic is based on the Bayes' theorem, which says your test results are, to some extent, determined in advance by your degree of likelihood for having the disease. I know this sounds complicated. Even first-year statistics students find it confusing. The theory points to a statistical probability: If you are at very low risk, you are more likely to have a falsely abnormal result. It's a very important principle that doctors use for any test we order to make a diagnosis, whether that's for heart disease, to look for abnormalities during pregnancies, or even to test for HIV.

I've seen younger women in my practice who have had stress tests as part of a company physical. They come in worried about their "positive" results. When I tell them they don't have heart disease, and that the test was wrong, they're extremely grateful. They say I "saved their lives." Truly, I did nothing. I just wish they had avoided the grief and hadn't done the test in the first place!

Stress Echo

A stress echocardiogram is a type of stress test involving an ultrasound of the heart. In this test, you will use a treadmill or stationary bicycle (the "stress" part), then move over to a table for an "echo," which takes ultrasound pictures of the heart. During the echo test, you'll get ultrasound jelly on your chest, and the technician will use a probe to look at your heart in several positions. The ultrasound usually takes around 30 minutes and carries no risk, although at times it can be a little uncomfortable if pressure is applied on the ultrasound probe in order to obtain better pictures. This is similar to an ultrasound that pregnant women receive except we are looking at the heart.

If you have a blood-flow problem to your heart, then with

stress, the heart will not move well. An ultrasound can pick up the motion of the heart—doctors call this wall motion. If there is a wall-motion abnormality at stress that is not seen at rest, this implies an area of the heart is at risk because there's a lack of blood flow.

Your doctor looks at a stress echocardiogram to see if your heart-muscle function is affected with chest pain and exertion. The stress echo complements a regular stress test. Unlike the stress ECG, the stress echo can visualize an area of impaired blood flow to your heart.

The success of a stress echo depends on the quality of the pictures. If you are very overweight, or if the lab doing the stress echo is not a high-volume or accredited lab, the information from the test may not be accurate.

Nuclear Perfusion Scan

Perfusion means "blood flow," so a nuclear perfusion scan takes pictures of blood flow to the heart, both at stress and at rest. In a nuclear perfusion scan, a technician will inject a radioactive chemical, or tracer, into your vein to follow the blood flow that goes to your heart. By observing the dye, doctors are able to locate which part of the heart may be lacking in blood flow. If you have a narrowing of blood flow to your heart, there will be less blood flow to your heart at stress (when you're exerting yourself) than there is at rest. In other words, the supply of blood will be less than the demand.

If you look at the heart as cross-sectional slices, each slice resembles the shape of a donut. During a nuclear perfusion scan, we take pictures of the slices when the heart is resting and also during stress. We then compare the scans. Under normal conditions, the slices look the same at rest and stress. However, if there's a problem with blood flow to your heart, then it looks as if a bite has been taken out of the donut. How abnormal, or "bitten," these images look helps doctors determine the problem.

A perfusion scan will reveal the abnormal blood flow, even if you don't have chest pain during the test or your ECG is normal. Doctors also order a scan to add information to the findings of an ECG or stress test. You often need the scan if you do *not* have a normal ECG result at baseline (during resting conditions).

A nuclear perfusion scan is not invasive and can be performed on most patients. The downside is you are exposed to a relatively small amount of radiation—roughly the equivalent of 10 chest X-rays. This amount of radiation is, by and large, considered low and comparable to the natural radiation we get by simply living our lives over about a two-year period. Having said that, I do not order nuclear stress tests on young people since they have a lifetime of exposure ahead of them—in contrast to middle-aged or older people. A young person will be exposed to more accumulative radiation over the years—whether it's from medical tests, from travelling in airplanes or from other sources. In principle, I won't order the nuclear perfusion scan lightly. I believe you should not have any scan of the body unless you are having symptoms.

If you're having a nuclear scan, you can be given an intravenous drug called Persantine to simulate exercise without truly stressing the heart. Persantine vasodilates, or opens up, the coronary arteries and diverts blood flow from the diseased artery to the healthy artery. The scan will show the relative difference in blood flow. Persantine may trigger nausea, headache or a transient sensation of chest pain. To relieve these symptoms, doctors may give you a dose of aminophylline, essentially a caffeine-based drug. Before you have a Persantine scan, you have to be caffeine free for at least a day so it can work properly.

Coronary Angiogram

A coronary angiogram is an invasive test to measure blood flow to your heart. It's the gold standard of testing to see if you have narrowings or blockages in your arteries. *Angio* means blood vessel, and *gram* means picture; a coronary angiogram means a picture of the heart's blood vessels, or coronary arteries. The benefit of a coronary angiogram is that it is the most definitive test doctors have, whereas the non-invasive tests such as stress tests and stress echos may not give doctors all the answers.

Here's how it works: After local freezing, a cardiologist will make a small incision in your leg or arm and insert a tube into your femoral (leg) or radial (arm) artery. The tube will then travel up to the heart through the aorta. You will have dye squirted into your coronary arteries. A technician will take X-rays of the arteries. There's low risk associated with dye. Talk to your doctor first if you suspect you may have a dye allergy. Your doctor may give you a medication such as Gravol or steroids to prevent an allergic reaction before the angiogram.

Tens of thousands of Canadians undergo coronary angiograms every year. However, because the procedure is invasive, there is a risk inherent in inserting tubes so close to the heart. Therefore, I don't recommend a coronary angiogram for everyone. Three in 1,000 patients receiving an angiogram may experience a life-threatening issue such as a heart attack or stroke. The tube might "tickle" your heart, causing an arrhythmia (see Chapter 9). The tube might even dissect, or tear, a coronary artery. On the other hand, 997 people out of those 1,000 will not have a problem. The odds are in your favour.

Another risk of an angiogram involves bleeding at the puncture site, where the tube enters your body, whether it's in the area of the leg (femoral) artery or arm (radial) artery. With a femoral puncture, there is a 1 in 200 risk of bleeding in the groin. The risk is slightly higher if you're overweight.

Many patients living with chronic kidney dysfunction also have heart disease. If you are one of these patients, your cardiologist will work closely with your kidney specialist (nephrologist) to treat you. One frequent area of concern, for instance, is that dye used in a coronary angiogram can cause harm to the kidneys. This applies only if you have severe kidney disease.

You'll be awake when an angiogram is performed, or perhaps on a sedative such as Valium to calm your nerves. You'll be asked to hold your breath from time to time as the dye is injected and X-rays are taken. When you have an angiogram, you're exposed to the equivalent of just over 10 X-rays' worth of radiation. Again, that particular radiation dose and your lifetime risk of radiation exposure are weighed against the benefit of dealing with a serious coronary problem.

I don't routinely send patients for angiograms if their hearts are generally stable. However, I will send patients for angiograms if they have an abnormal stress test or a worrisome scan. An angiogram is a necessary step to determine if you need to restore blood flow to your heart with either an angioplasty or bypass surgery (see Chapter 10).

After a heart attack, many (but not all) of you may need to receive angiograms as part of a program of quality care. You should be especially mindful of this if you are a woman. According to research, women are less likely than men to have this procedure. The reasons are not entirely clear. Women are often older and frailer when they have heart attacks. This may deter some physicians from putting them through an invasive angiogram. However, after a heart attack, women are often also at greater risk of having future heart problems. If you or a family member has had a heart attack recently and has not had a subsequent angiogram, talk to your doctor and ask: Why not? You don't always need to have an angiogram after a heart attack, particularly if you've done well on a treadmill stress test and have had normal nuclear perfusion scans or stress echos. However, it's better to ask the question.

Ultimately, it's important to have a (non-confrontational!) friend, family member or advocate accompany you to see the doctor, in order to help you ask informed questions. Undergoing tests can be nerve-racking if you don't have a basic but clear sense of the medical processes involved. By asking the right questions and being informed, you and your doctors can turn trepidation into reassurance. This applies whether you're in an emergency situation where a great deal seems to be happening at once or in a specialist's office where your time is limited.

We've just reviewed six of the most common tools for evaluation of coronary heart disease. However, they aren't the only tests you may have. Cardiologists rely on a variety of other screenings and measurements, whether it's for coronary artery disease or for non-coronary issues such as rhythm problems of the heart. Your doctors will determine the appropriate assessments depending on your symptoms and history. We'll explore several additional tests and their uses in the next chapter.

7

OTHER IMPORTANT TESTS FOR THE HEART

"If I have a heart-rhythm problem, what tests do I need to take and what will they reveal?"

In Chapter 6, we reviewed the key tests physicians use to evaluate your chest pain—including electrocardiograms, stress tests and blood screens. These are tests used to diagnose coronary heart disease, the blood-flow problems of the heart. Using a variety of other screenings, doctors can assess non-coronary heart problems as well. For example, they can evaluate how well your heart muscle is squeezing, or the efficiency of the heart's pumping ability (ejection fraction; see Chapter 1). We can look at rhythm abnormalities (arrhythmias) or assess the severity of murmurs, the sound caused when there is abnormal blood flow through the heart valve. For every issue with the heart, there are appropriate and sophisticated tools to measure and assess them. Here are detailed explanations of nine more investigations used in cardiology.

Echocardiogram

A transthoracic echocardiogram (or TTE), simply known as an echocardiogram, is a non-invasive ultrasound test. This scan allows doctors to take pictures of the heart valves and blood flow and to see how well your heart muscle is squeezing. For most heart problems, cardiologists usually need to evaluate your heart-muscle function using an echo.

We've already looked at a stress echo (Chapter 6). That's an evaluation of your heart at stress—you exercise on a treadmill and undergo the ultrasound. If you have a blood-flow problem to your heart, then with stress, the heart will not move well. The echo is able to look at the motion of the heart, which doctors call wall motion. A wall-motion abnormality at stress may put you at risk of a heart attack.

An echocardiogram isn't always used to assess the heart at stress, however. Mostly, it's used for a variety of other reasons. They're useful if you have valve problems or your doctor wants to rule out the possibility of a valve problem. For example, your doctor may have heard a murmur in your heart using a stethoscope during a physical exam. (You will read more on murmurs in Chapter 9.) An echo can determine if a murmur is serious or what we call innocent. An innocent murmur is when blood flows rapidly or abnormally in the heart because of, for instance, anemia or pregnancy. A serious murmur, on the other hand, can be an indication that there's a problem with your heart valve. An echocardiogram will help doctors make the diagnosis.

There are also things the test will not do. For instance, an echo will *not* determine if chest pain is actually coming from your heart. However, if you have had a heart attack and you have heart-muscle damage as a result, then an echo will pick up an abnormality in one of the walls of the heart at rest. We call this a regional wall-motion abnormality.

Sometimes, doctors need specific information and more precise pictures of the heart—for example, if we're planning surgery to repair (instead of replace) a mitral valve, the valve between the left atrium and the left ventricle. In this particular case, you may need a transesophageal echo (TEE). The heart sits very close to your esophagus. An ultrasound probe inserted into your esophagus towards the stomach may result in clearer pictures than a standard echo. The TEE test is very similar to a gastroscope, in which a tube is inserted through your mouth and into the esophagus in order to take pictures of the stomach, except that instead of having a light at the end of the scope, there is an ultrasound probe. You will not usually need a TEE unless you have complex valve problems.

MUGA Scan

MUGA stands for multi-gated acquisition. A MUGA scan is also called a radionuclide angiogram, or RNA. It's a scan of the heart that gives doctors specific information on how well the pump is functioning. MUGA is the gold standard of testing to assess your ejection fraction, which doctors need to measure to determine if you have heart failure.

We measure the ejection fraction (or EF) to determine how efficiently your heart is pumping blood. Think of your heart as a cup holding blood. The normal heart will eject—or pump—half of that blood forward with every beat. This amount is called the ejection fraction. Your ejection fraction will be reduced if the heart muscle is weakened and the pump is struggling. A normal EF is in the range of 55% to 70%. A low EF is less than 55%. A very low EF (under 30%) is a serious problem.

A MUGA is a nuclear scan, meaning that doctors use radioactive substances (dyes) to "see" how a particular part of the body is structured and functioning. MUGA scans assess the function of the left and, sometimes, right ventricles of the heart. When radioactive particles are injected into your bloodstream, they attach to your red blood cells. Doctors can detect the amount of red blood cells in your heart because there's "visible" radiation attached to them. The amount of cells is measured both when the heart squeezes and relaxes. This information is used to calculate your ejection fraction.

A MUGA study does *not* give us information about your valves or blood flow to your heart. Doctors use the test to assess patients who have weak heart-muscle function, either after a heart attack or because of certain chemotherapy treatments. MUGA is also a test if you have cardiomyopathy, a serious but rare case of a weakened heart muscle (see Chapter 9). The information the scan provides can determine whether your heart function is so impaired that you need therapies such as an internal defibrillator (see Chapter 11).

MRI

You may be familiar with MRI, which stands for magnetic resonance imaging. Perhaps you've had an MRI because of an injury to a part of your body, whether it's your back or your knee, or because you have had persistent headaches and your doctor wanted a scan of your brain. In an MRI procedure, a patient lies flat and is moved inside a large circular device that contains a powerful magnet. The magnet is used to create images of the human body.

MRIs are commonly performed in medicine. That said, it takes a particular set of circumstances for a heart MRI to be useful. In particular, you must lie still for a prolonged period of time. Otherwise, the picture can blur. Also, if your heart is beating too fast, the MRI won't give a clear image. So you must have a low heart rate for the test to be useful.

An MRI of the heart can take up to an hour to perform and is used in special conditions in cardiology. It can be useful, but it's not a test doctors will routinely order. It may be better at detecting unusual tumours of the heart, congenital abnormalities of the heart or rare conditions in which fat infiltrates the heart, or to determine if and where heart muscle is viable, or alive, after a heart attack.

Because of the magnets, you can't have an MRI if you have big pieces of metal in your body. Coronary stent inserts (see Chapter 10), on the other hand, are almost always safe in MRIs. Just check with the doctor performing the test to be sure.

PET Scan

A PET scan, or positron emission tomography, is a nuclear scan that looks at the activity of cells. Like all nuclear scans, it uses radiation to form a picture. It's often used in oncology to detect cancerous tumours and clustering of active cancerous cells in your body. In cardiology, it is sometimes used to see if your heart muscle cells are alive. That is, you may have had a heart attack, and your doctor is concerned about the extent of heart-muscle death, or inactive cells. A PET scan can determine if cells are still viable, or alive. Your doctor may need to assess this viability if you have a weakened heart muscle from multiple heart attacks and are being considered for bypass surgery or angioplasty (see Chapter 10). But a PET scan is not a routine test. These scans are usually reserved for patients with severe heart-muscle dysfunction—that is, an ejection fraction lower than 30%.

CT Coronary Angiogram

A CT (computed tomography) coronary angiogram is a non-invasive scan of your coronary arteries. With CT imaging, a technician will insert a dye into your veins. The technician will be able to trace the dye and produce detailed images of your blood vessels. The CT angiogram can also pick up calcium in your arteries—a sign of atherosclerosis—as well as assess narrowing in the arteries that supply blood to your heart. Keep in mind that these arteries are actually quite small; as a result, this imaging technique has come into use only in the last few years with the advent of sharper, more up-to-date scanners.

CT is often useful to identify complex issues such as a splitting or dissection of the aorta in the chest. This is considered a cardiac emergency. However, doctors don't always use CT angiography to provide an image of the heart. In other words, CT is not a first-line or routine test for screening you for coronary disease, mainly because of the radiation exposure involved in making a scan. A CT scan is also not as good as a more invasive coronary angiogram in terms of seeing any blockages in your arteries (see Chapter 6). The test exposes you to as much radiation as approximately 100 chest X-rays, but these levels are generally considered safe.

If you are obese, you will need a larger dose of radiation in order to see good pictures with CT imaging. That's one reason I tend not to routinely use CT angiography in my practice.

The radiation levels in a cardiac CT angiogram vary widely depending on the facility where the procedure is performed, who performs the procedure and the actual make of the machine.[1] This is a concern because high levels of radiation over our lifetimes are linked to the risk of developing cancer. Medical imaging is one of the largest sources of radiation we receive. Luckily, times have changed, and scans and technology now provide good images with lower amounts of radiation. Doctors are also aware of the issues and don't radiate people willy-nilly. When my father was a child, it was normal for a clerk in a shoe store to measure his foot with a form of radiation called fluoroscopy. The science of such tests is rapidly changing—and in the future, techniques may emerge to minimize the radiation doses further.

Holter Test

A Holter is a monitor that measures the rhythm of your heart. Your doctor may put a Holter monitor on you if you've been fainting and the concern is that it might be due to an abnormal heartbeat. The monitor will then look at how fast or slow your heart is beating over a day or two. During a Holter test, you are hooked up to electrocardiogram electrodes that are then attached to a tape recorder–type machine. A Holter monitor will assess all your heartbeats during the period of time it is worn, usually 24 to 48 hours. During this test, you are given instructions to press a button if you feel palpitations so that we can see the exact time of your symptoms and determine if they are due to arrhythmia.

Loop Monitor

A loop monitor is similar to a Holter but is worn for an extended period of time, usually two weeks. It monitors your heartbeat and stores only relevant data during that time—in other words, it will record any occurrences of arrhythmia. If you have an episode of palpitations, for instance, it can be recorded, stored and transmitted over a telephone to a central data analysis area. Since many patients do not have palpitations or fainting episodes on a daily basis, a loop monitor is a good test for assessing symptoms over a longer time span. Loop monitors are also useful tests to look for episodes of atrial fibrillation, a condition of irregular heartbeats that occurs in roughly 5% of people over the age of 65 (see Chapter 11).

ABI Vascular Doppler

The ABI, or ankle–brachial index, is a test for circulation problems that can put you at risk of heart attack or stroke. Poor circulation in your legs is almost always due to atherosclerosis, the same disease where plaque accumulates, narrowing the arteries that supply blood to your heart. If you have circulation issues, you'll often have difficulty walking, cramps or leg fatigue (see Chapter 5).

The ABI is essentially a comparison of the blood pressure measurement in your legs (measured at the ankle) and the blood pressure in your arms (the brachial measurement). Under normal circumstances, when there's no narrowing in the vessels, these measurements will be the same. However, when you have atherosclerosis in your legs, the pressure there will be lower than the pressure in the arms. Doctors need a special technique to hear the blood pressure in your legs: It's a Doppler ultrasound, a piece of equipment that's placed on the foot.

> If you or a loved one has an ABI of less than 0.9, you are at a markedly higher risk of dying than if you don't have peripheral arterial disease—otherwise known as PAD, or artery disease of the legs (see Chapter 8). Patients with low ABIs and PAD are six times more likely to die from heart attack or stroke than the general population.

Patients who have severe quality-of-life issues with circulation-related cramps in their legs (claudication; see Chapter 5) may require angioplasty of the legs or even bypass surgery of the legs. In this case, a Doppler ultrasound is useful to pinpoint where the narrowings and blockages are. If symptoms are not severe, the treatment is to stop smoking and to take medication to lower your blood pressure and your cholesterol. You may also require Aspirin-like medications to help thin the blood and prevent clots from forming. You will have to reduce any other risk factors for vascular disease.

Coronary Artery Calcium Scores

A healthy artery is one that is calcium free. However, calcium may build up in arteries that are diseased with atherosclerosis, which leads to heart attack and stroke. A CT coronary artery calcium score is a measurement of calcium in your arteries. It does not directly tell you if you have coronary artery disease, but the more calcium you have, the greater you are at risk. It's not routinely used as a screening tool because of the inherent exposure to radiation from the scan.

In the old days before advanced testing such as angiograms and CT scans, one of the tests used to assess coronary disease was a special X-ray (fluoroscope) that looked for calcium in your arteries. This is no longer done. Our technology has evolved, and we have better ways of looking at the heart.

A coronary calcium score doesn't give doctors much additional information if you're at low risk for future heart disease (that is, your risk of having a heart attack or stroke in the next 10 years is less than 10%). It also won't add valuable information if we already know you have many risk factors or you already have heart or vascular disease. It's the group of people in the middle—if you're at moderate risk—that might benefit from the findings of a calcium test. For example, it may sway the decision to go on cholesterol pills.

Coronary artery calcium scoring has become very popular in the United States and in areas of for-profit medicine. If you search the Internet, you'll find many websites touting the virtues of this technique. Every year in my Toronto practice, I see people who have come back from Buffalo having paid hundreds of dollars for a coronary artery calcium test or even a total body CT scan. This makes entirely no sense to me. As a preventive cardiologist, I believe you're much better off looking at your risk factors and summing them up with a global risk assessment (see Chapter 2). It also makes no sense when people with diabetes, hypertension or chronic kidney disease seek additional test results to tell them what we already know—that they are at risk! If you are already at high risk for heart disease, more tests won't tell you otherwise.

Personally, I'm not a fan of coronary artery calcium scores and do not recommend the test for my patients. Exposing you to radiation and looking for calcium is not an ideal way to assess your risk.

❤ You need to know: What will each of the tests diagnose?

- **Tests used to diagnose and manage coronary artery disease include ECG, blood tests, stress test, echocardiogram, nuclear perfusion scan, CT, PET and coronary angiogram.**
- **Tests used to diagnose rhythm problems of the heart include ECG, Holter monitor and loop monitor.**
- **Tests used to diagnose congestive heart failure include ECG, echocardiogram and MUGA.**
- **Tests used to diagnose valve problems include echocardiogram and ECG.**
- **Tests used to diagnose peripheral arterial disease include ABI.**

The Limits of Testing

In reality, very few medical tests can show a definite picture of whether or not you have heart disease. One exception is the angiogram (see Chapter 6), which looks directly at the arteries. However, an angiogram is an invasive test, carries some risk and is not recommended for everyone with stable heart disease. In contrast, stress tests and scans give indirect evidence for coronary heart disease, meaning there's a reasonable amount of proof to support an inference that you have the disease. Also, when doctors take your risk prediction score, it's to determine your *future risk* rather than to give you a yes/no answer to the question "Do I have heart disease now?"

It's entirely possible that if you are at high risk of having cardiovascular events in the next 10 years, you may have some early development of atherosclerosis. However, unless your arteries have been narrowed by 50% or more, you are not going to have symptoms now. If your doctor already knows you are at high risk, then it doesn't really matter if a test shows you have either a 20% or a 40% narrowing in your coronary arteries. This is because your doctor's focus will be the same in either case: reducing your risk of artery disease and heart attacks with lifestyle changes and medications.

On a weekly basis, patients ask me which tests can "see" the blockages in their arteries. If you have heart disease, you may want to visualize that plaque is "shrinking" in your coronary arteries as proof that your doctor is doing a good job. But your cardiologist doesn't always need to see a picture to determine if your treatment is working. Yes, there is a test called IVUS (intravascular ultrasound). It's primarily a research tool, and it's not routinely performed in clinical care. Recent IVUS studies have shown that very high doses of cholesterol-lowering medications will cause plaque in the arteries to regress, or shrink.[2] But a study like this is not that relevant to your care. To treat you, doctors rely instead on research from clinical trials. These trials show if a medication or treatment is effective at reducing actual "events"—whether that's reducing hospital admissions for angina or heart attacks and strokes. In large clinical trials, cholesterol-lowering medications have been proven to reduce a patient's risk for future heart attack and stroke. That's far more important than a test to "see" how much actual plaque, or junk, you have in your coronary arteries. A picture may be worth 1,000 words—but not necessarily in preventive cardiology.

8

WHAT YOUR DIAGNOSIS MEANS: CORONARY HEART DISEASE

"I've just had all the tests, and they confirm I've had a heart attack. What does that mean for me now?"

If you have been diagnosed with heart disease, it can feel like a devastating blow, especially if your doctors tell you your condition is serious. You may be facing a future that seems, for now, overwhelming. Maybe you're confronting the prospect of surgery, or you're worrying that you may no longer lead the life you once did. On the other hand, diagnosis is a step in the right direction—and many of you will feel a certain relief to know what exactly you're dealing with. After all the testing, waiting and anxiety, a diagnosis means you're closer to getting the treatments and tools you need to manage and live with your disease. To begin with, you need to know what the actual diagnosis implies—what *is* the disease, what causes it and what lies in your immediate future?

Before we answer these questions, remember there is a wide spectrum of diseases of the heart and blood vessels. *Cardiovascular disease* is the umbrella term for all heart problems. Cardiovascular diseases are further divided into two subsections: coronary and non-coronary.

We've spent the majority of this book covering the former: the risk factors, symptoms and testing for coronary heart disease (CHD), alternately known as coronary artery disease. CHD refers to the plumbing problems of the heart, or the narrowing of the coronary arteries caused by atherosclerosis. If the arteries are narrowed and the heart does not receive enough blood, the heart pump will be starved of essential nutrients and oxygen. It will not function properly. This could lead to angina (chest pain) or a heart attack. In general, coronary problems are the ones doctors talk about when we use the shorthand "heart disease." Needless to say, coronary heart disease can be life threatening. Let's deal with each coronary condition in detail.

Stable Angina

If you have been diagnosed with angina, that means you've experienced pain in the chest that occurs when your heart is not receiving enough blood. As a doctor, I always use the words *chest pain* in describing angina, but in fact, angina is not usually a jabbing or stabbing. It's not a pinpoint kind of pain. Angina is a deeper sensation of discomfort, often a squeezing or heaviness in the chest. Angina can be felt anywhere from the chest into the arms, jaw, back, shoulder blades or even teeth. It's usually reproducibly exertional—that is, the discomfort comes on with activity and is relieved with rest, and you can bring it on if you push yourself.

Under times of increased stress, such as when you are physically active or emotionally upset, your heart has an increased demand for blood. If you have atherosclerosis, or a buildup of plaque in the arteries, the blood supply is compromised, and the heart will not receive the supply it requires. This supply–demand mismatch causes angina. You typically won't feel the pain if you're resting because the heart needs less blood and can cope with the flow, even with atherosclerosis.

If your doctor says you have stable angina, this means you have a pattern of angina symptoms that have not changed over time. Usually, this means your discomfort appears with emotional or physical activity and lasts for a few minutes during every episode of angina; you can relieve the pain, which is a pressure, squeezing or tightening in the chest, with rest or a dose of nitroglycerine, a spray or tablet medication that helps open up the arteries. Angina is often accompanied by a shortness of breath. The discomfort can start in your chest but can radiate into your throat, arm, jaw or back. Stable angina doesn't usually occur when you're inactive, out of the blue. But you may also feel the pain in cold weather—which constricts blood vessels—or after you've walked up an incline.

If your angina appears more frequently, or comes on at a lower exertional threshold than before, it means blood flow to the heart has been suddenly disrupted and reduced further, and your angina may no longer be stable.

Unstable Angina

If you have angina that lasts for a prolonged or unusual period of time, say 20 minutes, it could be unstable. You should seek emergency medical attention if your angina is not relieved with rest or two sprays of nitroglycerine five minutes apart, starting at five minutes into the discomfort. With unstable angina, you might feel cold and clammy, look ashen or grey, or feel nauseous. Most telling of all, the chest, arm, throat or jaw discomfort that you usually experience only with exertion starts to appear at rest, wakes you up from sleep or occurs at a lower threshold of activity. This is usually a warning sign that there's been a progressive and potentially serious narrowing in the blood flow to your heart. In other words, it's a signal that your body is *trying* to have a heart attack.

Ironically, a blood clot is the result of a good idea gone bad. Our bodies are designed to heal when blood vessels are broken; forming a blood clot under healthy and normal circumstances is important to prevent bleeding. However, when a clot forms inside an artery wall, it can be life threatening.

With unstable angina, some of the atherosclerotic plaque in your artery may have ruptured. It may start flapping around in your artery wall. This ruptured plaque is, figuratively, a magnet for blood platelets to gather and form a blood clot. A blood clot in the artery wall can lead to a heart attack.

As we'll cover in greater detail later on in the book, the treatment for unstable angina includes many forms of intravenous, injected or oral blood thinners, given in hospital to settle your blood platelets and prevent a blood clot from forming. Some forms of unstable angina may be treated solely with medication in hospital; others require more serious intervention such as angioplasty or even, rarely, open-heart surgery (see Chapter 10).

Heart Attack, or Myocardial Infarction

A myocardial infarction means, bluntly, heart-muscle death. However, not all heart attacks are as severe or cause as much heart-muscle damage as they used to decades ago. Medical technology has advanced; so too has patient awareness about coronary disease and heart attacks. Compared with generations ago, these days more people are aware of the symptoms of heart attacks and therefore know to seek emergency care when they're experiencing chest or arm pain.

A heart attack occurs when a blood clot forms in your vessel wall, often because the plaque has become unstable and the blood flow in that area is fully disrupted. This may lead to a large, severe heart attack. At other times, a blood clot can try to form, but the disruption to the blood flow is intermittent and eventually settles down, not causing severe damage.

Doctors have become very sophisticated about checking for heart-muscle damage, which is done by looking for abnormalities in blood tests (cardiac enzymes) and by charting a specific

Anatomy of a Heart Attack

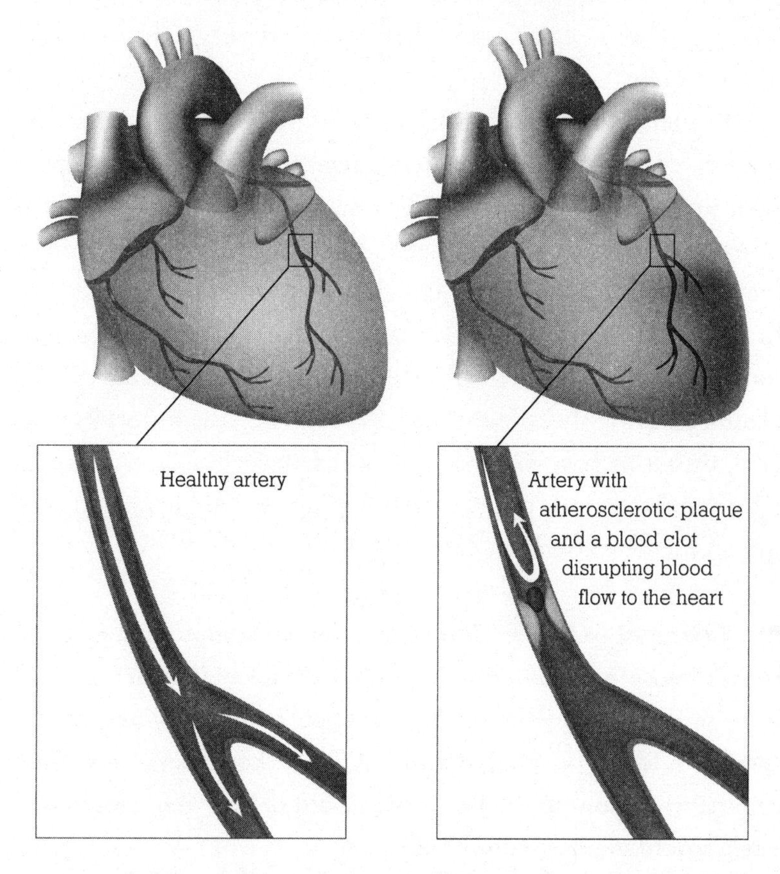

pattern of changes in an electrocardiogram (see Chapter 6). You can be labelled as having had a heart attack even if blood tests show a small amount of microscopic damage to the muscle. When a heart-muscle cell is damaged, it can leak a substance called an enzyme (whereas healthy cells keep their contents inside). Doctors are able to detect this leakage even in cases of minor damage, involving only a few heart-muscle cells (myocytes).

Damage will result in an abnormal blood test. Note that this is very different from having a full-fledged blood clot in your artery, causing chest pain that is continuous for hours and hours. If you do not seek medical attention early enough after experiencing prolonged chest pain, you can have a heart attack that leaves you with significant heart-muscle damage. The damage is permanent.

The term for the spectrum of heart attacks is *acute coronary syndrome* (ACS). Essentially, ACS ranges from patients coming in with unstable angina that settles down to massive "Hollywood" heart attacks—the kind you see in the movies. That's a common and classic case of a patient clutching the chest, being unable to breathe. I can't stress enough that if you or a loved one has prolonged chest discomfort, especially associated with feeling cold or clammy, having shortness of breath or having discomfort in your arm, throat or jaw, you should stop whatever it is you're doing, whether that's work or grocery shopping or child care, and seek urgent medical attention—call 9-1-1.

❤ **You need to know: The most common symptom of a heart attack for both women and men is chest discomfort. If you have prolonged discomfort in your chest, especially associated with feeling cold or clammy, having shortness of breath or having discomfort in your arm, throat or jaw, you should seek urgent medical attention.**

When you're diagnosed with a heart attack, doctors will act quickly to treat you. We'll spend more time describing how and why in Chapter 10, but here are the highlights: If a clot is completely blocking your artery, and this usually occurs suddenly, then physicians will use clot-busting medications (thrombolytic therapy), or they'll perform an angioplasty. The latter is a procedure in which a balloon on the tip of a catheter is inserted into your coronary artery and then opened up to get rid of the narrowing where the clot formed, thus restoring blood flow to your heart. Quite often, patients are also put on intravenous blood thinners around the time of a heart attack in order to reduce the likelihood of a clot recurring.

In my business, I say time is heart muscle. Every minute counts. If you're treated within six hours of a heart attack, there's a good chance you'll minimize the damage. After six hours, the damage is hard to repair. Keep in mind that it takes time even when you are *in* the hospital to prep for receiving an angioplasty.

One of my patients is a man in his 40s who did shift work at a job he loved. He was so worried he might lose his job that he reported for duty even as he was having major discomfort in his chest. It turned out to be a heart attack that resulted in serious damage to his heart muscle. Although he is now managing his heart disease with medications, lifestyle changes and cardiac rehab, the experience has left him with anxiety. He's now so nervous about his condition that he seeks help for every little twinge he feels. If he had put himself first when he had his original chest pain, he wouldn't be dealing with the additional emotional stress of living with heart disease and a damaged heart muscle.

When blood flow is disrupted to the heart muscle during a heart attack, your heart can become "irritable," which usually means you are at risk of developing a life-threatening arrhythmia (often a fast heartbeat). In these cases, patients need to be in an emergency room in order to be resuscitated, or shocked out of the arrhythmia with a defibrillator. In some situations, the heart can become irritable and slow down to the point of a heart block. In this case, patients may need a temporary pacemaker surgically inserted while they are having an acute heart attack. Obviously, this has to be performed with speed and urgency at a hospital, where you can receive high-tech, advanced care as the heart attack is unfolding.

❤ You need to know: During a heart attack, you may also experience life-threatening arrhythmia because your heart is not receiving enough blood flow. If you're not already at the hospital, call an ambulance!

When the heart muscle dies from a heart attack, the area is inflamed and can be prone to rhythm problems later on. In time, often a scar (fibrosis) forms. A large scar on the heart is fertile ground for further complications. Chiefly, you can develop a short-circuit in the electrical system, leading to serious rhythm problems, or malignant arrhythmias. (In fact, you might need an implantable defibrillator to prevent this very thing, if you've been left with significant heart-muscle damage after a heart attack.) Malignant arrhythmias can be suddenly and mercilessly fatal—yet another reason to call an ambulance when you're having chest pain rather than drive yourself to the hospital. Emergency medical teams are equipped to deal with very serious arrhythmias.

❤ You need to know: It's crucial that if you're having a heart attack, you do not drive to the hospital. Call 9-1-1 for an ambulance. EMS teams are equipped to deal with time-sensitive, life-threatening arrhythmias.

After the acute treatment of heart attack, it's very important to receive the proper longer-range therapies and medications. We'll cover these in Chapter 14.

Chest Pain and Normal Coronary Arteries

Sometimes, a patient can appear to be having classic angina pain, but when all the tests are done, the cause is undetermined. This means there are no detected blockages or narrowings in the arteries. This is more often the case in women than in men and is usually clarified when doctors examine the heart with a coronary angiogram. One name doctors give to this extensively evaluated syndrome is chest pain and normal coronary arteries. We also call the condition cardiac syndrome X. Why *X?* Because we don't know what causes it. There's a host of unproven theories as to why syndrome X occurs and various proposed treatments—many of which do not work.

Some say syndrome X is caused by a miscommunication from overly sensitive receptors (mechanoreceptors) in the muscle of the heart, which send signals that, ultimately, the brain registers as pain. Sometimes the pain is due to musculoskeletal or gastrointestinal issues. Other times, patients are under high stress, whether it's because of a fear of dying from a medical condition, as a family member did, or because they've just gone through the anniversary of the death of a loved one. For others, merely walking into a hospital can bring on chest pains. In rare cases, I've cared for patients who have endured an underlying emotional trauma. That's not to say that all patients with chest pain and normal coronary arteries have psychological issues—to the contrary. It's quite frustrating for patients who have this kind of mysterious but genuine pain. Often they are bright, well adjusted and highly functional in their careers and home life. The syndrome X label tends to be overused for patients, especially women. We don't know why this is the case. I don't like labelling patients or, worse, dismissing their pain. The good news is that many of my patients with chest pain and normal coronary arteries get better with time.

If you are diagnosed with this syndrome, your doctor should advise you to adopt a heart-healthy diet and lifestyle, address any stress factors in your life and, when appropriate, begin a trial of antidepressants and/or stomach medication. Working on your quality of life and heart disease risk factors will make you feel better about your health and helps minimize the pain.

Peripheral Arterial Disease

PAD (formerly called peripheral vascular disease) is a serious condition that is often underdiagnosed, under-recognized and undertreated. If you have this disease, it means you are at significantly increased risk of having a heart attack or stroke. With PAD, your arteries are narrowed by atherosclerosis in various places in the body other than the heart. The disease primarily appears in the legs. The symptom of PAD is claudication, which is, essentially, angina of the legs. If your blood flow is restricted in the legs as opposed to the heart, instead of having chest pain when you exert yourself, you'll have leg pain. PAD traditionally appears as a cramp in the back of the calf that's relieved after you sit down and rest. Sometimes, however, PAD is asymptomatic—that is, you have the disease but don't have symptoms.

❤ **You need to know: If you have blood vessel disease in your legs, you may feel fatigue or pain in the legs when you walk because your legs are not receiving enough blood. You're also at risk of heart attack and stroke: If you have atherosclerosis in your legs, you're likely to have it in your heart and in the blood vessels of the neck.**

In North America and Europe, an estimated 27 million people live with peripheral arterial disease. Almost half of these individuals are asymptomatic, meaning they don't experience any of the signs of the disease. Although there is little data available on PAD in Canada, the disease likely affects approximately 4% of the population over 40.[1]

I think of PAD as a poor cousin of cardiovascular disease because it's not as "glamorous" an issue or as well discussed in the public as heart attack and stroke, but it's just as deadly. If you have blood vessel disease in your legs, that's a marker for atherosclerosis elsewhere in the body. In fact, if you have PAD, you are six times more likely to die from heart attack or stroke than the general population.

The risk factors for coronary heart disease are generally similar to those for PAD. In other words, you are at risk for PAD if you have diabetes, elevated cholesterol and high blood pressure and if you smoke or lead a sedentary lifestyle. It's crucial that people be aware of signs and symptoms of PAD and that family doctors ask and screen for the disease. PAD is diagnosed using a straightforward test called an ABI or via vascular Doppler ultrasounds (see Chapter 7). There are some risk factors that are more common for developing PAD than coronary artery disease. Patients who have PAD are more likely to be smokers or have diabetes.

As a cardiologist, I'm passionate about the PAD cause, so much so that I've been involved with the Canadian Cardiovascular Society in writing guidelines on PAD for physicians. Treatment for PAD involves the same risk-reduction strategies for preventing coronary heart disease—among them eating well, being active, stopping smoking and reducing hypertension and bad cholesterol. Find out more information on the disease via the National Heart Lung and Blood Institute (www.nhlbi.nih.gov) and the PAD Coalition (www.padcoalition.org).

The good news is you can reduce your risk by eating healthily, exercising and, most importantly, stopping smoking, in addition to taking cholesterol-lowering medications. Patients with PAD may also take Aspirin-like medications or antiplatelet drugs to help prevent clots from forming.

If you have PAD, you are encouraged to "walk to pain"—actually pushing yourself to develop pain in your legs will improve your exercise tolerance. That's an important distinction between PAD and coronary heart disease; if you have heart disease, you shouldn't try to walk to bring on chest pain. There's also some evidence that walking helps people with PAD develop new blood vessels in the legs, or "natural bypasses." Their exercise tolerance improves with time without putting them at risk of leg attacks. In some situations, patients with PAD may not be able to walk at all. If your quality of life is compromised because of atherosclerosis in the legs, then your doctors may suggest a leg angioplasty or leg bypass surgery to help open up the affected blood vessels, in addition to cholesterol or Aspirin-like medication. Remember, angioplasty is a "quick fix"; it does not treat the disease—which is atherosclerosis.

9

WHAT YOUR DIAGNOSIS MEANS: NON-CORONARY HEART DISEASE

"If I'm having palpitations, does this mean I'm about to have a heart attack?"

Arrhythmias—or rhythm disturbances of the heart, which include palpitations—can be daunting for even the most medically informed patients. I have a friend who has years of training as a nurse (and is married to a physician). She was experiencing palpitations and came to see me, worried sick that something was very wrong with her heart. Of course, it's understandable that if you feel your heart is pounding out of your chest, you may become overtaken with concerns. However, in this case, her palpitations were benign, or not serious. Arrhythmias range in severity, but my friend was experiencing a common, non-serious kind of palpitation. I was also able to reassure her with a simple fact: People with arrhythmia are generally not at risk for developing the more serious coronary heart diseases such as atherosclerosis, which can lead to angina, heart attack or stroke.

Arrhythmia is part of a spectrum of non-coronary heart diseases. If you are diagnosed with a non-coronary heart disease, then your condition is not related to the plumbing and the blood vessels of the heart. Rather, your heart could be failing, or its rhythm could be disturbed, for reasons other than blood flow. The issues may be congenital, meaning they were present at birth. Whether or not these conditions are dangerous depends on the specifics of your situation and the nature of the disease.

Types of Arrhythmia

Arrhythmia can range from not serious to life threatening. If you have an arrhythmia, you may have extra beats, missed beats, a fast heart rate or a slow heart rate. These electrical disturbances of the heart bring a range of symptoms. You may not sense anything at all, or you might feel palpitations and vigorous heartbeats. An arrhythmia can even cause you to pass out.

If you have a common, non-serious arrhythmia, your heart may simply be predisposed to having an extra beat and then pause, but your heart won't stop. After the pause, it's normal for the heart to contract vigorously with the subsequent beat. The pause itself creates a moment for blood to fill in the ventricle (the heart's main pumping chamber). This is often what patients feel—a vigorous contraction from a heart full of blood, after the initial extra beat.

As a cardiologist, I determine the severity of an arrhythmia by asking two questions: First, is the heart otherwise normal? I'm looking to rule out heart-muscle damage often caused by coronary heart disease or valve problems. If there's no structural heart disease—that is, the pump and the valves are functioning well—the arrhythmia is usually not a serious concern.

❤ **You need to know: Arrhythmia is usually not a serious condition if you have a structurally normal heart—meaning the pump, ejection fraction and valves are working as they should. If your heart fits this description and you're feeling extra beats, don't let your arrhythmia worry you.**

Question number two: Is there hemodynamic compromise? Meaning, is there an inadequate amount of blood getting to the brain? Lack of blood to the brain is worrisome and leads to lightheadedness or fainting. The appropriate therapy for this condition depends on whether the fainting is related to a heart beating too slowly (bradycardia) or too quickly (tachycardia).

Let's elaborate on each of these rhythm disturbances.

Slow rhythms, or bradycardia, occur when electrical impulses are blocked as they try to pass from one part of the heart to another. When you faint because your heart is beating too slowly, or there is a complete heart block, it means the top part of your heart (the atria) is sending electrical signals that are blocked before they reach the bottom part of your heart (the ventricles). In other words, the top and bottom parts of the heart are not "talking" to each other. If you faint because of a very slow heart rate, you may need to have a pacemaker surgically implanted—that's a device that stimulates the electrical activity of the heart and regulates the heartbeat (see Chapter 11).

In contrast, the heart can beat too fast. Fast rhythms originate from electrical problems either in the top of the heart (supraventricular tachycardia, or SVT) or the bottom of the heart (ventricular tachycardia).

Supraventricular Tachycardia

SVT means there's an electrical problem, causing a fast heartbeat, in the top of the heart. SVT is a general term that applies to a group of rhythm disorders. The most common is a short-circuit called atrioventricular nodal re-entry tachycardia (AVNRT). In an otherwise normal heart, the electrical impulse in your heart would start at the top of the SA node and travel down to the AV node and then to the ventricle. But with AVNRT, there is a short-circuit in electrical conduction through the AV node, which causes the heart to beat fast. Many otherwise healthy people are born with this condition, which is treated either with medications to slow the impulse in the short-circuit or by an ablation, a procedure using a catheter, that eliminates the short-circuit. SVT is easily treated and does not put you at risk for future coronary heart disease. Sometimes SVT does not need medical treatment at all.

❤ **You need to know: Supraventricular tachycardia (SVT), a fast rhythm that originates in the top of your heart, is a common problem in otherwise healthy people. It's usually easily treated and does not put you at risk for future coronary heart disease.**

A supraventricular tachycardia is usually not a serious issue; however, fast rhythms such as atrial fibrillation, atrial flutter, ventricular tachycardia and ventricular fibrillation are far more serious. Let's discuss them one by one.

Atrial Fibrillation

Atrial fibrillation, or A-fib, is a type of specific SVT that requires significant attention. It occurs when the upper chamber of your heart beats irregularly in a disorganized manner. If I were to listen to a heart with atrial fibrillation, I would not hear the normal, steady "lub dub" pattern of the beating. Some patients can noticeably sense the irregularity; others may not.

Atrial fibrillation occurs in roughly 1% of the general population. The risk increases the older you are: Approximately 4% of people age 60 and older and nearly 10% of the population age 80 and older have atrial fibrillation.[1] High blood pressure also increases the risk. This is because hypertension creates increased pressure in the left ventricle of the heart, which then creates a pressure buildup that may cause your atrium to stretch. When your left atrium is enlarged, there is a greater chance that it may beat irregularly.

Normal Rhythm vs. Atrial Fibrillation

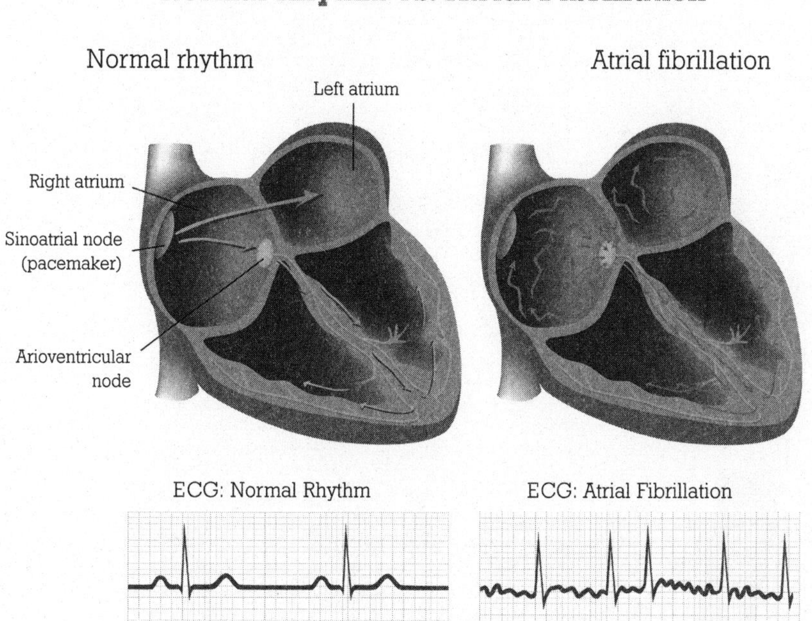

People who have either an overactive thyroid (hyperthyroidism) or an underactive thyroid (hypothyroidism) may experience atrial fibrillation because the thyroid is the thermostat in the body. When it's out of whack, your heart may beat irregularly. There's also an association between alcohol intake and atrial fibrillation. In med school, I learned about the "holiday heart syndrome," where people would arrive in the emergency room in atrial fibrillation after binge drinking over a long weekend or festive holiday. I saw a young woman in my practice with such a problem—she didn't need heart medication, but she had to stop drinking. Other causes of atrial fibrillation include sleep apnea and mitral valvular disease—when the mitral valve on the left side of your heart is not working as it should. (See page 176 for more on valve problems.) If you have a new diagnosis of atrial fibrillation, your doctor will order an echocardiogram to rule out the possibility of serious valve problems.

Atrial Fibrillation and Stroke

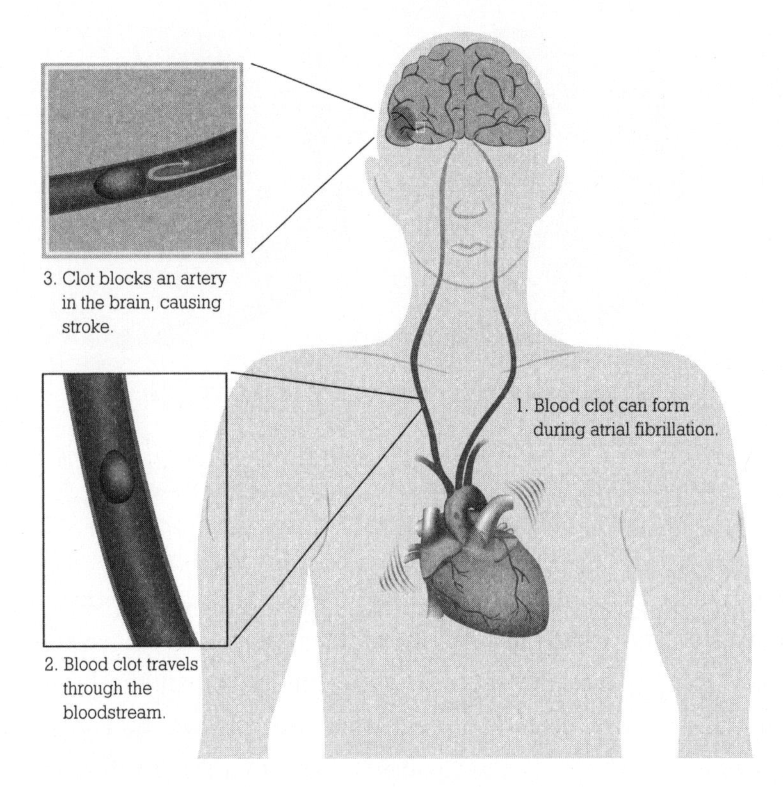

One of the potentially serious consequences of atrial fibrillation is that blood clots may form in the atrium, the top part of the heart. The clots may travel through the heart to the aorta and blood vessels in the brain, disrupting the blood's flow and causing stroke (a "brain attack").

Atrial Flutter

As with atrial fibrillation, atrial flutter is a serious type of SVT—an irregularity at the top part of the heart that puts certain patients at risk for stroke. The difference is that in atrial flutter, the irregularity is more organized in its activity. This short-circuit can be more easily treated with a modern procedure called an ablation (see Chapter 11).

Ventricular Tachycardia

Otherwise known as VT, ventricular tachycardia is a condition in which rapid heartbeats start in the ventricles in the bottom part of your heart. In most cases, VT is a serious, or malignant, arrhythmia that requires important treatments. However, the severity of VT depends on the company it keeps. In other words, if you experience episodes of light-headedness caused by VT, and your condition is accompanied by heart-muscle damage from a previous heart attack, your doctor will likely recommend implanting a defibrillator, a device that can shock the heart out of this rhythm. The weaker your heart muscle, the more susceptible it is to serious, malignant arrhythmias. You can have a cardiac arrest—the heart can stop—as a result of a fast heart rhythm such as ventricular tachycardia. When this occurs, a shock from either an external or internal defibrillator can save your life.

Ventricular Fibrillation

This is one of the most serious rhythm problems you can have. It is a disorganized, fast rhythm coming from the bottom part of the heart. The heart doesn't pump when it goes into V-fib. Ventricular fibrillation is also associated with a sudden loss of blood flow, so it can occur during a heart attack. Ventricular fibrillation is a common cause of cardiac arrest.

To find out how doctors treat these arrhythmias, see Chapter 11.

Congestive Heart Failure

The term *congestive heart failure* (CHF or, simply, HF) may sound terrifying, but it does not mean you are destined to die imminently. If you have heart failure, your heart muscle is not working normally. It is either weak or stiff and cannot pump blood effectively through the body. Let's expand on this: generally, congestive heart failure is caused by either a stiff but normally squeezing heart muscle (called diastolic dysfunction) or a weakened heart muscle (systolic dysfunction). Either case will result in a buildup of pressure and fluid in the lungs, which causes shortness of breath that is usually worse when you're lying down and better when you're sitting up. A classic history of someone with congestive heart failure is being short of breath upon lying down at night to sleep. Patients with congestive heart failure may also find themselves needing to sleep propped up on extra pillows because that's the best position they can find at night for breathing. Often patients will wake up gasping for air, and they will try to open windows to feel relief.

When your heart muscle doesn't pump efficiently, the heart sends signals to your brain. Your brain then transmits signals to the rest of your body, instructing it to retain salt and water, which causes swelling. When the left side of your heart doesn't work well, pressure and fluid back up in the lungs and then the right side of your heart. The fluid will build up in the veins of your body. If a significant amount of fluid has accumulated, then there will be swelling in your legs.

To diagnose heart failure, your physician will perform a physical exam that includes feeling the heart through your chest, listening to your heart, listening to the lungs and looking at the

Congestive heart failure is a common and serious problem affecting millions of people all over the world every year. More than 400,000 Canadians have survived heart attacks or other serious cardiac issues and are living with heart failure. The Heart and Stroke Foundation provides an excellent guide for these survivors called *Managing Congestive Heart Failure* (download it from www.heartandstroke.ca).

veins in your neck that are connected to your heart. It's vital to assess vein pressure—called jugular venous pressure, or JVP. That's essentially the "fuel gauge" that indirectly measures the pressure on the right side of your heart and lungs.

We will also look for swelling of the ankles. The type of swelling, or edema, that may be due to heart failure is called pitting edema because when you push your finger on the swelling, a mark or pit is made that takes some time to resolve. This will also be seen if tight socks or shoes are worn in the area of the swelling. This swelling is different from other, often non-serious, causes of swelling that people experience.

As we touched on in Chapters 6 and 7, tests to determine congestive heart failure include electrocardiogram (ECG), echocardiogram, chest X-ray and blood tests. Doctors perform an ECG to see if your heart muscle has become thick or weak because of a previous heart attack. Often, patients who have severely weak heart muscles will have an abnormality that appears in testing called a left bundle branch block (LBBB). An echocardiogram, or ultrasound of the heart, is also used to determine if the heart muscle is enlarged, stiff and thick, or weakened from a heart attack, or if heart failure is caused by a narrowed or leaky heart valve.

With the chest X-ray, doctors are looking for fluid in your lungs. However, if you have scarring on your lungs or lung disease for other medical reasons (such as smoking), it may be difficult to determine how much fluid actually exists. It may also be hard for your physician to determine if your shortness of breath is a result of heart failure or from non-heart-related causes such as chronic obstructive pulmonary disease (COPD, the other name for emphysema and chronic bronchitis) or asthma. That's why doctors are starting to use a blood test for N-terminal brain natriuretic peptide (or NTBNP), a chemical in the blood that is increased in patients with heart failure. It's not necessarily ordered, however, if you have severe fluid on the lungs (pulmonary edema) and the diagnosis is obvious to your doctors. (For treatments of congestive heart failure, see Chapter 12.)

Heart Failure After a Heart Attack

When the heart doesn't work, your blood pressure falls and blood and vital fluids aren't pumped forward into your body. Instead, they back up into your lungs. This life-threatening consequence of a heart attack is called cardiogenic shock. The chances of cardiogenic shock being fatal are high. You are more likely to go into shock when you have an extremely large heart attack or if you seek medical attention too late in the game.

The treatment for cardiogenic shock requires an urgent transfer to a heart catheterization lab for emergency treatment such as angioplasty. Not every hospital has such a facility. If you are ever in the situation where a family member is in shock in the emergency room, be proactive and ask when they will be transferred to a cath lab for an angioplasty. There are studies showing that women are less likely to be transferred when in cardiogenic shock, just as they're less likely to go into intensive care.[2] The reasons aren't exactly clear-cut, but it's safe to say that, traditionally, physicians tend to undertreat women and underestimate their risk.

Being proactive and asking the right questions—even if it's "Is there anything else you can do? Can my mother be transferred to a hospital that performs angioplasty?"—can never hurt.

In some cases, you may experience temporary heart failure during a heart attack—but not cardiogenic shock. Even though this sounds like you escaped the worst, you're still at increased risk for developing future complications, especially if your heart muscle is damaged. If your heart-muscle function is very poor—for example, your heart's ejection fraction is less than 35%—you are at risk for developing future heart failure as well as arrhythmia. You may need to have further testing such as a stress test or coronary angiogram in order for doctors to assess the function of the heart and the extent of the damage. The MUGA test (see Chapter 7) is the gold standard for assessing your ejection fraction, which tells us how well your heart is pumping. If your ejection fraction is low (below 30%) and your heart failure has been controlled for more than six months, you may be a candidate for receiving an implantable defibrillator. On the other hand, if your ejection fraction is above 40% on the MUGA scan, a defibrillator is not usually warranted.

❤ You need to know: The most common cause of congestive heart failure is a weakened heart muscle from a heart attack. If you have poor heart-muscle function, you are at risk for developing heart failure as well as heart rhythm problems.

Cardiomyopathy

You may have heart-muscle problems that are not caused by heart attack. This is called cardiomyopathy, a serious but rare case of a weakened heart muscle. Non-ischemic cardiomyopathy is the term applied to severe heart-muscle dysfunction that's caused by certain viruses or other, sometimes undetectable, sources. Hypertrophic cardiomyopathy is a thickening of the heart muscle that can run in families—that is, it's genetic.

Two Types of Cardiomyopathy

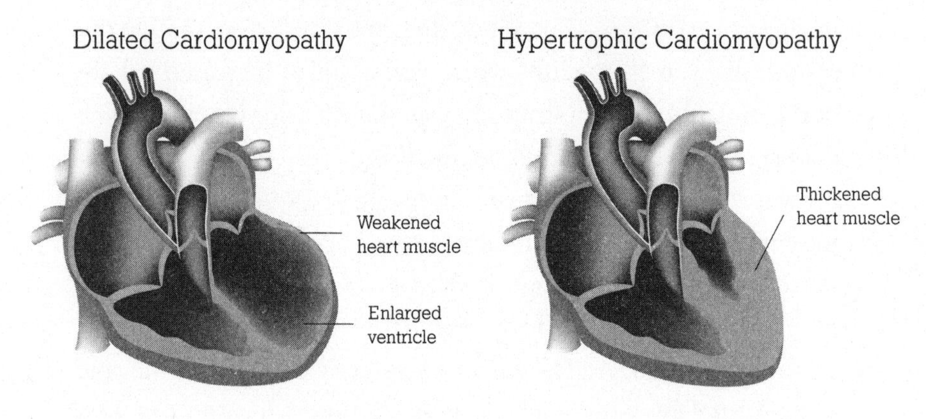

Scarily, your heart can "catch a flu," and you can be left with a severe deficiency in heart-muscle function. Cardiomyopathy may occur in pregnancy; the exact cause of this is unknown, but it's a serious condition that may show up in women after they've delivered a baby. In rare cases, cardiomyopathy can also be caused by toxicity from severe alcohol use as well as certain forms of chemotherapy. Although the research into the latter is new and evolving, there's some indication that some heart-muscle damage from chemotherapy is reversible. For instance, damage caused by newer breast cancer drugs such as Herceptin is proven to be more easily reversible than damage caused from other forms of anthracycline-based chemotherapy. Treating cardiomyopathy involves the use of medications and careful follow-up with a cardiac specialist, in addition to adoption of heart-healthy lifestyle changes.

In general, I tell patients with cardiomyopathy that with treatment, one-third of people will get better, one-third of people will stay the same, and one-third will have heart-muscle deterioration. Unfortunately, there is no clear way to predict if you will respond to the treatment or not.

Sometimes, the results can be surprising. I saw a 41-year-old patient who had a flu-like illness and had been diagnosed with cardiomyopathy. Although she was taking all the right medications, she remained so sick that doctors told her she might need a heart transplant. Six months later, she came into my care. To everyone's delight, we discovered that thanks to the correct medication and the tincture of time, her heart-muscle function had recovered completely. She was literally crying with joy when I told her she could go back to her normal routine. Her heart had healed.

Stiff Hearts in Women

Heart failure due to a stiff heart muscle is also called heart failure with preserved ejection fraction. The *preserved,* in this case, means there's a normal amount of blood being pumped forward by the heart; however, the heart doesn't relax and fill as well as it should, leading to a buildup of fluid in the lungs. This diastolic heart fail-

Left Ventricular Hypertrophy (A Cause of a Stiff Heart)

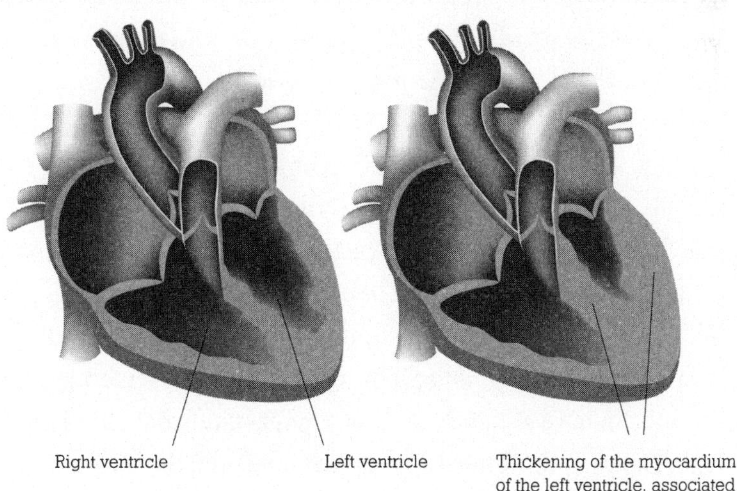

ure is more commonly seen in older women. It can also be seen in patients with diabetes or high blood pressure. You may live with this type of heart failure and not be aware of it because you don't have any symptoms and your body is able to compensate for the stiff heart. In these cases, you may often experience another problem, such as an irregular heartbeat due to atrial fibrillation. This could push you to develop symptoms of shortness of breath, leading to a diagnosis of a stiff heart and treatment for the condition.

Common Valve Problems

There are four valves in your heart. The two on the left side (the mitral and aortic) are the most likely to become narrow (stenotic) or leaky (regurgitant or insufficient). For every person I see with an actual serious valve problem, I see three more who are only led to believe they have one. These patients are sent to me after they take an echo test that reveals a mild abnormality in blood flow.

❤ You need to know: Sometimes modern medicine is *too* good. For instance, an echo test is so sensitive it might pick up patterns in blood flow that aren't really a cause for alarm. If you see the words *trace, physiologic* or *mild* on your valve report, there is usually no reason to worry.

One such case involved a 53-year-old woman who came in to see me, clutching her echocardiogram report, convinced that she was dying. The echo had indicated that the top part of her heart, the atrium, was enlarged and one of her valves had trace regurgitation, or leakiness. What she didn't know was that the reading was in fact in the normal range. This is a key point to remember: Every patient can have a slightly different range of normal—and the echo report that reads abnormal requires interpretation from a doctor. Keep this in mind the next time you review any results with your doctor. Our medical technology these days is very sensitive and will pick up things that aren't really a cause for alarm. Rest assured that when the echo report says "trace, physiologic or mild," there is usually no issue at all, and your valve is still in the acceptable range.

Murmurs

A murmur is an abnormality a doctor picks up with a stethoscope. It's caused by abnormal blood flow and sometimes, but not often, is associated with symptoms of shortness of breath and fatigue. A murmur could result from a narrowing (stenosis) or leakiness (regurgitation) of the valve. At other times, murmurs are innocent—not a result of an abnormal valve. In young women, anemia or lower hemoglobin counts can be innocent causes of a murmur.

Aortic Stenosis

A narrowed aortic valve is very common and is potentially a serious issue. It's seen in two different groups of patients: people in their 80s and patients in the 30 to 50 age range. The younger people are commonly born with an abnormal valve; the older people have wear and tear on the valve over time. There are no medications that can prevent or treat a narrowed valve. Rather, the valve has to be replaced in surgery. But generally we don't replace aortic valves unless the person is having symptoms such as shortness of breath, angina, light-headedness or fainting. If you or a family member has been diagnosed with a narrowed aortic valve, or aortic stenosis, and you have any of these symptoms, see your doctor immediately.

❤ **You need to know: Symptoms of a narrowed aortic valve include shortness of breath, chest pain, and light-headedness or fainting. If you have been diagnosed with aortic stenosis and you have any of these symptoms, see your doctor immediately. The treatment is surgical. The valve needs to be replaced.**

Approximately one in 100 people is born with a slightly abnormal aortic valve, meaning they have only two leaflets (cusps) in the valve instead of three. This bicuspid aortic valve works very well for many years but over time may see mechanical wear and tear, which can cause a scarring of the valve leaflet and a narrowing of the valve. Usually, this takes 30 or 40 years to occur so that if you were born with a bicuspid aortic valve, you usually won't see the effects of a narrow valve until you are nearing or in middle age.

Normal and Bicuspid Aortic Valves

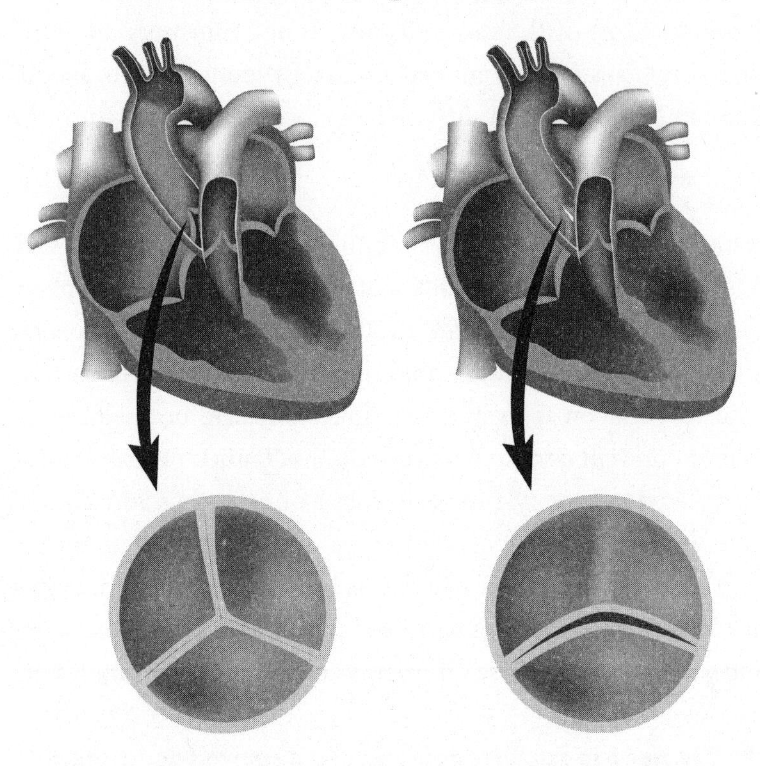

Normal aortic valve   Bicuspid aortic valve

The rest of the population isn't immune to wear and tear of their normal, tri-leaflet aortic valves. We're all living longer lives, and mechanical deterioration is not uncommon in the elderly. I often see highly functional individuals in their late 70s and 80s who present with symptoms and a severely narrowed aortic valve. Valve replacement, which is open-heart surgery, has significant risks. Still, even in many older people, the risks are outweighed by benefits. If you have a very elderly family member with aortic stenosis, you may wish to discuss his comfort level with surgery early on, when the valve is not too narrow. Would he want major open-heart surgery at the age of 86 or not? Discuss the risks and rewards with your doctor even before you get sick and need surgery.

Aortic stenosis, although often picked up by hearing a murmur on exam, can also present for the first time with congestive heart failure. If you have a very narrowed valve (or tight aortic stenosis) and symptoms of heart failure, angina or fainting, there is a 50% chance you might die within a year if the valve is not replaced. On the other hand, if you have the same severe narrowing of the aortic valve but no symptoms, your outlook is better. We usually do not operate on an aortic valve unless it is very narrowed *and* you are having symptoms. I see some patients who don't show any symptoms, years after they've been diagnosed with aortic stenosis. The most important course of action is that once a diagnosis is made, the patient is followed carefully over time.

Lately, a new technique has emerged for replacing the aortic valve that does not require an extensive open-heart surgery. It's called transcatheter aortic valve implantation (TAVI; see Chapter 16 for more). This technique is being evaluated in patients who have no other options—usually frail, very elderly individuals. One of my patients is an 88-year-old veteran and long-time key figure in his hometown. He had open-heart surgery (bypasses) 15 years before I met him. However, since his bypasses, his aortic valve narrowed gradually to the point of aortic stenosis. As a person with severe aortic stenosis, his quality of life was drastically impaired. He was also at risk of not surviving the condition within a year of diagnosis. At his age, the risk of redoing heart surgery would be too high. But he was a good candidate for a TAVI procedure, which he underwent successfully. The change was significant. Before his TAVI, he had been in hospital for a month or so at a time—too ill to go home. But only a month after the procedure, he was well enough to lay a wreath at the Remembrance Day memorial in his local town, as he had done for years. He's now living his 89th year, feeling more vigorous than I could have ever imagined.

Doctors measure the amount of stenosis, or narrowing, of an aortic valve in two ways: We calculate the valve area and measure the pressure gradient across the valve. In other words, if you have an obstruction to flow, there will be a pressure buildup before that obstruction. In general, a very narrowed aortic valve is considered a valve of less than 1 cm^2 or with a gradient greater than 40 mm Hg. Think of it this way instead: A narrow aortic valve is one that measures less than 1.2 cm^2, or the size of a nickel. The valve will continue to narrow by 0.1 cm per year on average. If you or a family member has been found to have a narrowed aortic valve of 1.5 cm^2, six may not need an operation for another five years or so. Everybody progresses at slightly different rates.

Aortic Regurgitation

Aortic regurgitation is a leaking aortic valve, a less common condition than aortic stenosis. It can occur from an infection of the valve, during which the valve is damaged, or if you have an abnormal valve, which can wear down over time, causing it to leak. If your aortic regurgitation is chronic, meaning it's gradual over time, this is often treated with medication such as water pills (diuretics). If the aortic valve is leaky, more blood will flow back into the left ventricle of the heart. With time, this excess load on your heart can cause it to enlarge. If you have severe aortic regurgitation, you need to be watched to ensure that your heart is not enlarging. An enlarged heart may mean your valve needs to be replaced in surgery, depending on your doctor's findings. If an aortic valve becomes leaky all of a sudden, because the valve has been damaged by infection, then your heart is less able to compensate and deal with the sudden excess blood. Acute aortic regurgitation, if it is severe, is a cardiac emergency requiring immediate surgery.

Mitral Stenosis

A narrowed mitral valve is known as mitral stenosis. It usually occurs if you had rheumatic fever as a child. It can cause a progressive buildup of pressures and backflow of blood in the lungs. Usually the symptoms develop gradually and are insidious. The stereotypical patient is a woman who can no longer walk up the stairs with her laundry and feels more tired over the course of a year. Although mitral stenosis is easily detected with an echo test (see Chapter 7), the condition is more difficult to diagnose because the symptoms tend to be vague. As well, the murmur is more difficult to hear when your doctor examines you.

You can live for many years with a narrowed mitral valve and not have any symptoms at all. However, if your valve narrows significantly, you can develop increased pressure in the lungs (pulmonary hypertension), which is serious and requires treatment. Some patients can be treated initially with medication such as water pills (diuretics). Other patients who have pulmonary hypertension will need the valve fixed. Narrowed mitral valves can often be repaired with a catheter procedure known as mitral valvuloplasty, which is performed in cath labs in specialized cardiac centres in North America. However, not everyone is an ideal candidate for a valvuloplasty. If your valve has lots of calcium, does not move well or is thickened significantly, your chances of a successful valvuloplasty are lower. You might need an open-heart valve replacement instead.

It's common to have calcium deposits over time in the mitral valve that do not cause an actual narrowing. This is called mitral annular calcification, or MAC. This is not a serious problem; however, if you need valve surgery for other reasons, the calcification around the base (or annulus) of the mitral valve can make the procedure more difficult to perform.

Mitral Regurgitation

Mitral regurgitation is a leaky mitral valve. A very leaky mitral valve can cause fluid and pressure to build up, creating serious problems such as high pressure in the lungs (pulmonary hypertension). Managing this serious problem depends on how leaky your valve is, as well as the cause of the leak in the first place. After a heart attack, sometimes the heart enlarges and stretches your mitral valve. The mitral valve will then become leaky as a secondary consequence of the heart-muscle enlargement. Secondary mitral regurgitation due to an enlarged heart is usually treated with medication (diuretics and ACE inhibitors) to take the pressure off your heart and lungs or open up (vasodilate) your arteries.

However, if your heart is not enlarged or damaged for another reason and the chief problem is the mitral valve itself, then the leakiness is called primary mitral regurgitation. If this is severe, in addition to medications, you may need surgery. The type of surgery depends on the problem at hand. Sometimes surgeons are able to repair your mitral valve, and other times your mitral valve needs to be replaced. A mitral valve replacement is a big operation, and cardiologists do not recommend it lightly (see Chapter 13).

Whether narrowed or leaky, mitral valve problems can be associated with serious heart rhythm conditions. Along with an increased pressure in the lungs, there is also a potential for increased pressure buildup in the left atrium of the heart, so you may experience rhythm problems such as atrial fibrillation (see Chapter 11).

Pericarditis

Pericarditis only feels serious and scary. In fact, this painful condition isn't perilous, and having had pericarditis in your lifetime does not increase your risk of future coronary heart disease.

Here's what it is: The pericardium is the sac that sits around your heart. It's an evolutionary leftover—it truly doesn't have a purpose in the body of a developed human. Sometimes the pericardium can become inflamed and irritated—called pericarditis—usually because of a virus such as a common cold. This usually passes, but in some instances, as white blood cells rush in to help heal the cold, fluid accumulates between the pericardium and the heart itself. The inflamed pericardium can come into contact with your heart and cause pain from friction. (The analogy is getting into a car in the summer and trying to slide across the hot leather seat.) This can result in severe, stabbing chest pains, which feel worse when you lie down since the fluid has time to accumulate in the lying position. The pain can be severe enough to prompt you to go to the emergency room. Pericarditis shows up as classic changes on the electrocardiogram (see Chapter 6). The treatment is usually a course of anti-inflammatory medications.

One of my patients is a young woman who had ongoing episodes of inflammation around the lining of her heart. Initially when this happened, she went to the emergency room, was seen by several physicians and was prescribed short courses of anti-inflammatory medications. But her symptoms kept returning. She was seen by my colleague, a rheumatologist, who specializes in looking for rare causes of inflammation. Fortunately, the patient did not have autoimmune diseases such as lupus. When I took her history, I found out that every time she went to the emergency room, she had two or three days of treatment and then stopped. That turned out to be the culprit. The appropriate treatment for pericarditis is usually six weeks of anti-inflammatory medication—even when your symptoms go away after a few days. It's vital to complete the full course of therapy.

Pericarditis often occurs in otherwise healthy young individuals and may reappear over time. Rarely, patients may need potent medications such as colchicine to prevent recurrent inflammation. If you have pericarditis, you need to be checked by your physician to ensure that the inflammation is not more extensive than in the sac around the heart.

Myocarditis

Myocarditis (*myo* for muscle, *card* for heart and *itis* for inflammation) is inflammation of the heart muscle. Think of it as the heart catching a very serious virus. In the last 100 years, during the great flu epidemics, myocarditis was a cause of death. Fortunately, this potentially fatal inflammation of the muscle is rare.

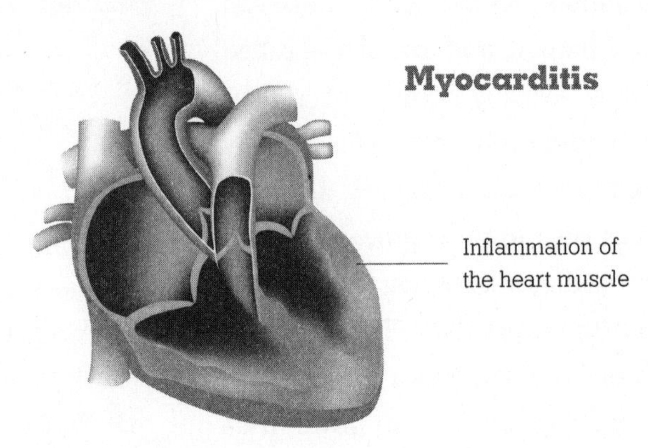

Myocarditis affects younger people, usually patients in their 40s. Most often, myocarditis is mild in nature, and the symptoms are usually non-specific and flu-like—including muscle aches, shortness of breath and fatigue. Fewer than 25% of patients with myocarditis will have a fever. When your heart muscle is inflamed and it's more serious, you might feel stabbing chest pain that is worse when lying down and better when sitting up. We diagnose myocarditis by ordering an electrocardiogram (ECG), doing blood tests and assessing the heart-muscle function with an echocardiogram (see Chapters 6 and 7).

Myocarditis is generally more serious than pericarditis because when the heart muscle is inflamed or irritated, you can experience arrhythmia or, in uncommon cases, your heart-muscle function may be affected. Myocarditis may also cause sudden cardiac death. *Fulminant myocarditis* is the term for a rare, severe and overwhelming inflammation of the heart muscle. Patients with fulminant myocarditis face life-threatening problems and should be assessed by cardiac specialists in specialized heart centres.

Myocarditis is not genetic. That is, if you have a family member who has had myocarditis, you are not more likely to be at risk of developing it, nor does having myocarditis as a younger person put you at risk for developing future coronary heart disease. Thankfully, many people with myocarditis survive, and their heart-muscle function *can* recover over time.

That's a positive note to end on as we reach the end of this chapter on non-cardiac issues. At this point, we've defined and detailed more than a dozen conditions related to the heart. There's an abundance of terminology to digest, I know, but it's valuable information to rely on, especially when you or a loved one has had an emergency heart problem or has been newly diagnosed, and there seems to be little time to pause and decode what is happening around you. Think of this information as a key to open the door to patient–doctor dialogue about your health and future prognosis, as well as a key to the rest of the book, which will answer the question you've been asking all along: "How will I get better?"

PART IV

Managing Your Heart Disease

10

TREATMENTS FOR CORONARY HEART DISEASE

"My wife had a heart attack at 63 and my brother had one at 55. She had surgery while he didn't. How do I know if they're getting the right care?"

To answer the question above, we have to look at the myriad facts relating to each situation. It isn't actually fair to compare the wife and the brother. There are so many individual details that determine the course of each person's treatment—how quickly they were seen by physicians when they had their heart attacks, the extent (if any) of heart-muscle damage, their overall health, the extent of atherosclerosis in their cardiovascular systems, and their other health issues and risk factors. Over time, doctors will look at how well they respond to interventions. In addition, the outcome in each case will be impacted by how motivated the individuals are to adopt heart-healthy habits and take their medications—for life!

Physicians know that the true practice of medicine is not cut and dry. Caring for a patient is as much an art as it is a science. That said, doctors rely on a series of sound guiding principles and a wealth of scientific research and medical practice to help inform their decisions. Let's flesh out the basics of treatment.

Risk vs. Benefit

One of the main principles of medicine is risk vs. benefit. The concept is that most of our therapies, drugs, surgeries and interventions have benefits in tandem with some form of risk. Generally, the risk is known and does not change from person to person. Risk, however, can change in certain groups, such as the elderly or very young. Anything that is done in medicine, from a treatment perspective, should have a risk-to-benefit ratio that favours the benefits. The basic math is apparent—we want to do more good than potential harm—but the equation is not always as clear as it seems.

Take the use of acetylsalicylic acid (ASA, commonly known as Aspirin). Many of you are aware that taking ASA regularly is good for your heart. It is. Specifically, ASA is considered an antiplatelet medication, meaning it will prevent platelets from sticking and causing a blood clot in your arteries. The research also reveals that if you have heart disease, ASA reduces your future risk of heart attack or stroke. But ASA can also cause bleeding. In most adults, the risk is small and the benefits are plentiful. On the other hand, there's no compelling reason for, say, a child to take a daily ASA. A child's risk of developing a heart attack in the near future is low. Yet a child's risk of bleeding with ASA is small but ongoing. Therefore, there is more risk than benefit for young people to take ASA to protect themselves from heart attack. This is an obvious example, but it helps you understand the concept of risk vs. benefit.

If you are older (in your 70s or 80s) and physically frail, you may be at higher risk of encountering complications, including stroke, during a procedure. However, you may benefit *more* from the procedure or interventions than a younger person, because your risk of future heart problems is greater. It's complicated! That's why you should see a specialist with years of training and a depth of experience to figure out the issues at hand.

❤ **You need to know: A risk-to-benefit ratio determines if a particular intervention or treatment is warranted, based on the premise that the treatment's benefit should far outweigh the risk. It's a nuanced science: Only an experienced specialist can accurately weigh risks and benefits for individual patients.**

The risk-to-benefit principle also applies to testing. For example, an angiogram (a test that visualizes blood flow) has a small amount of risk inherent in the procedure (see Chapter 6). Generally if you have just had a heart attack, I often recommend an angiogram. However, if you are well and without symptoms, you are unlikely to benefit from having an angiogram. What's more, an angiogram shouldn't be used to tell doctors what they already know. I often have patients who come in and ask for multiple tests, but if the test is not likely to add information or change my management of their condition, then it will not lead to better care for the patient. Sometimes it's more important to listen to what a patient is saying, deal with the exact question, and sort the issue out with a history, physical exam and simple testing.

Medications: The ABCs of Managing Heart Disease

If you've had a heart attack, or have been diagnosed with coronary heart disease, you need to take specific medications to help reduce your risk of future problems with your heart. In fact, most of my patients living with heart disease need to be on several medications daily—and forever—even if they've had an angioplasty or coronary surgery. Medications are an essential part of your care because they *treat the disease.* Surgeries and high-tech procedures, on the other hand, are a quick fix. Of all the vital drug therapies, the "big three" are antiplatelet medications, cholesterol medications (statins) and ACE inhibitors. Most people with coronary heart disease need to be on all three.

It's important to understand that many of the drugs we use in cardiology do not make you feel better; rather, they make you live longer. Classic examples of these are the cholesterol-lowering statin drugs and blood pressure medications. You won't necessarily "feel" the effects of these drugs—and you certainly won't feel or see what you are preventing. But the medications are working to extend your life in a way that's imperceptible to you.

❤ **You need to know: Ask your physician, "Will this drug make me live longer or feel better—or both?" It's very useful information for focusing your expectations as a cardiac patient.**

All the therapies and treatments for coronary heart disease work just as well for women as they do for men. But alarmingly, women are simply not receiving all the medical interventions that physicians have at their disposal. According to a recent study,[1] North American women are less likely than men to be on cholesterol medications a year after a heart attack. The reasons are unclear. There may be a "patient factor"—that is, women are less keen to take medication than men—or it may be that women are less likely to be prescribed medications or that they feel more side effects than men and therefore stop taking their medications.

I'll tell you a story that still sends chills down my spine. One spring day not too long ago, I saw a patient for the first time who had been diagnosed with atrial fibrillation—a serious arrhythmia, or rhythm disturbance, of the heart. She is a "young" 65-year-old who is active, is gregarious and was just starting to enjoy her retirement from a rewarding career. This woman has a history of hypertension and atrial fibrillation (see Chapter 9), which, in combination with her age, put her at increased risk of a stroke. Worried about this risk, I prescribed her a blood-thinning medication. Unbeknownst to me, she did not fill her prescription. About six weeks later, she was at her cottage with her husband, having never taken the medication. According to her husband, she was standing on the shore while he was swimming in the lake. He remembers looking up for a moment only to see her fall down—collapsed on the dock. They were in the middle of nowhere, 90 minutes from a hospital, and she had had a massive stroke. If only she had taken her pills, this tragic incident could have been prevented. Miraculously, my patient didn't die. Her brain has recovered to an impressive extent, but she now walks with a cane and is traumatized by her decision regarding her medication.

You may have heard of a reaction called the Hawthorne effect. It occurs when a subject improves his behaviour, without necessarily trying to do so, simply because he is being evaluated or studied. I think there's an element of the Hawthorne effect when a patient asks a doctor a series of relevant questions. The doctor becomes more attuned to the patient's needs. Asking the right questions is critical in ensuring that you or your loved one is receiving the right care. The question may be as simple as "Is my father or mother on the right medication after a heart attack, and is there anything else you might suggest?" You don't need to know medical specifics to make your health care provider think about the important issues.

There's a moral to every story, and the moral of this one is simple: If you are living with heart disease, coronary or otherwise, talk to your doctor and make sure you're on the right medications. If you're not, ask why! Asking the right questions will empower you. And please, please, fill your prescriptions and take your meds as directed.

Beyond drug therapy, of course, one crucial aspect of treating heart disease is lifestyle modification. Reducing the risk factors of heart disease before you have any kind of heart problem at all is called primary prevention (see Chapter 4). Secondary prevention refers to preventing heart problems *after* you have been diagnosed (see Chapter 14). By and large, for coronary heart disease, primary and secondary preventive measures are similar. The difference is that the stakes are higher once you receive a diagnosis. With secondary prevention, the payoff is also more rewarding—making changes can have a substantial effect in reducing your risk of a recurrent heart attack or stroke.

If you have had a heart attack or know somebody living with heart disease, you're likely more motivated to make a lifestyle change—or at least you should be. We know that maintaining a healthier body weight, being more active and exercising regularly, as well as eating a healthier diet lower in fat, can help you or your family member live longer (see Chapter 4).

To keep it all in focus, here is a list of the main treatment imperatives—from medications to prevention steps.

A

Antiplatelet medications: In general, all patients with coronary heart disease need Aspirin-like medication to prevent the platelets in the blood from sticking and causing a clot in a diseased artery. The big question cardiologists ask is, what dose and type should a patient receive? Within the first year after a heart attack, many patients are on dual (meaning two) medications. The most common dual antiplatelet medication used after a heart attack is a combination of clopidogrel and ASA. Newer effective drugs are also being evaluated. How long you need to take these newer drugs is up for debate. You usually need to be on ASA for life if you have heart disease, but you may be on dual antiplatelet therapy for only one year, depending on various issues after a heart attack or angioplasty.

ACE inhibitors: Angiotensin-converting enzyme inhibitors are a group of medications for blood pressure that have also been tested in patients with coronary heart disease. ACE inhibitors affect a hormonal system in the body called the renin angiotensin system. Specifically, the medication curbs the production of a substance in the body that can raise your blood pressure. ACE inhibitors can also benefit the health of your blood vessels and, if you are diagnosed with coronary heart disease, will help reduce your risk of heart attack and stroke. When I put a patient on an ACE inhibitor after a heart attack, I am essentially prescribing a blood pressure pill for reasons other than blood pressure control. If you have heart disease, these drugs have been shown to reduce the likelihood of a recurrent heart attack, regardless of your blood pressure.

ARBs: This acronym stands for angiotensin II receptor blockers. They are an alternative medication for patients who can't tolerate ACE inhibitors. Sometimes patients taking ACE inhibitors will develop a dry, hacking cough. If this is the case, their doctor may switch them to ARBs, which are useful in reducing future heart problems. That said, ACE inhibitors are the first choice in medication when it comes to protecting your blood vessels.

B

Beta blockers: These drugs can help you live longer with coronary heart disease because they block the rush of adrenalin to the heart and slow your pulse. If you have heart-muscle damage and are at risk for congestive heart failure, blocking adrenalin to your heart is a good thing to do; a low resting pulse rate protects your heart from physical stress. If you've had a significant heart attack, beta blockers help reduce your heart's irritability and lower your risk for developing a life-threatening arrhythmia. Beta blockers have also been proven to reduce death rates of patients with congestive heart failure. I often prescribe beta blockers to patients with angina because it allows them to run around and engage in activity without concern that their hearts will begin to race. In the past, beta blockers came with a list of bothersome side effects, including fatigue, sexual dysfunction and severe asthma. Fortunately, the newer beta blockers that have emerged on the market are less likely to cause these problems. The majority of my patients—including individuals with asthma—tolerate this type of drug, though sometimes younger patients may develop fatigue on the medication. After a heart attack, some of you may experience a loss of interest in sex and intimacy for psychological reasons, not because of your drugs. The most common side effect of a beta blocker is no side effect at all.

Blood pressure control: It's vitally important to manage your blood pressure if you have had a heart attack or have coronary heart disease. Some medications prescribed for your heart can also affect your blood pressure; others are primarily blood pressure pills that may also affect your heart rate and heart-muscle function. It sounds complicated, but there are medications prescribed specifically for your heart that can also lower your blood pressure, and there are blood pressure pills that can help regulate your heart rate and affect heart-muscle function. Determining which blood pressure medications are right for you is a decision your physician will make individually, based on your situation. It's important to know that if you are on blood pressure medications, you should not stop taking them just because you are "feeling" fine. Believe it or not, this happens all the time. Blood pressure medications are usually meant to be taken for life—unless you make dramatic lifestyle changes (see Chapter 4).

C

Cholesterol treatment: It's essential to know that if you have coronary heart disease, you should be on a cholesterol medication, even if your cholesterol is normal and you lead a healthy life. Many large randomized trials show that statin medication reduces the future risk of heart attack, stroke and overall survival—even if your cholesterol level is fine.

Again, most of my patients with heart disease are on this medication for life. I understand it's disheartening for them to hear this news, and often I'll re-evaluate their medication plan every three to five years. But in more than two decades in the practice of medicine, I've found no data to dissuade me from keeping my patients on ongoing cholesterol-lowering drugs. The benefits outweigh the risks.

That said, patients on cholesterol medications need to have their blood checked at least annually to monitor liver function and a muscle enzyme called creatine kinase (CK). Millions of patients on these drugs will have no abnormalities detected in the blood work. What's more, any abnormality that may emerge is almost always reversible. Some patients will complain of muscle aches, but this is the exception to the rule. If you have muscle aches on one type of cholesterol medication, you may not have aches on another similar drug. Given the benefits, it's worth trying either a lower dose or a different medication within the same class of drug. Recently, there's been concern that certain cholesterol medications may slightly increase your risk of developing diabetes.[2] Although that may be true, the benefit from these cholesterol drugs far outweighs the risk.

Cigarette cessation: If you have heart disease and are a smoker, the best risk-reduction strategy you can take is to quit. People who smoke have twice the risk of having a future heart attack after an angioplasty or bypass surgery than non-smokers.[3] Of course, stopping is always easier said than done. Quitting smoking is *a process,* not an event, and most smokers will need several attempts before they succeed. Ask your doctor for strategies to help you become smoke free.

Doctors used to believe that nicotine replacement—a stimulant—was dangerous to give to people even in hospital, but studies on smoking cessation now suggest otherwise. If you continue to smoke after a heart attack, with each puff you take, high levels of nicotine will quickly be released into the bloodstream. However, if you are given a nicotine patch, then the release of nicotine is slower and more gradual. The nicotine is released into your veins rather than arteries, so it's safer. Believe it or not, I've seen patients leave the coronary care unit to go for a smoke. This is why we use nicotine replacement in hospital. It's better than the alternative.

How exactly do you stop smoking? You can look for help—whether you're picking up smoking-cessation pamphlets or engaging in group or individual therapy. Drugs are also useful. Most studies suggest the best way to quit smoking is with a combination of supportive counselling and drug intervention.[4]

As I mentioned earlier in the book, newer smoking-cessation medications such as varenicline (sold as Champix in Canada) are considered safe for outpatients living with coronary heart disease. Studies are underway to look at the safety of these drugs for patients with recent heart attacks—on that point, the jury is still out.

❤ You need to know: Most studies suggest that the best way to quit smoking is with a combination of supportive counselling and drug intervention.

Cease hormone replacement therapy (HRT): As I wrote earlier in this book, hormone replacement therapy will not turn back the clock and make women younger, nor will it reduce their risk of heart disease. In fact, taking estrogen and progesterone may cause the blood to become thicker and may lead to clots. The American Heart Association recommends that women stop HRT for a year after a heart attack.[5] The problem is that some women with coronary heart disease also have severe symptoms of menopause. I've seen several women with both conditions in my practice, and I have to weigh risk vs. benefit in order to advise them. Overall, it's my opinion that if you have had a heart attack *and* you're having *severe* uncontrollable symptoms of menopause, you may wish to accept a small risk of staying on the hormone replacement therapy as long as you are on cholesterol medications (statins) at a reasonably high dose. However, it's not a convincing argument to say you want to continue HRT simply because it makes your skin look better or you just feel more youthful. Having mild menopause symptoms is not a valid reason to stay on hormones after a heart attack, either.

D

Diabetes control: Managing diabetes is almost as important as quitting smoking. We know that when your blood sugar is high, your risk for developing atherosclerosis increases. If you have heart disease and don't do a good job controlling your diabetes, you are at greater risk for a future heart attack, stroke and even death. Talk to your doctor about the particulars of diabetes control, or visit the website of the Heart and Stroke Foundation (www.heartandstroke.ca) or the Canadian Diabetes Association (www.diabetes.ca) for more information.

Diet: A heart-healthy diet is essential if you are living with heart disease, whether or not you have diabetes or are on medications to control cholesterol and blood pressure. Try to maintain a healthy body weight, eat lower-fat foods and read nutrition labels with a view to avoiding high fat and sodium. (See Chapter 4 for more information.)

E

Exercise and education: Anyone who has a heart attack, bypass surgery or angioplasty should be sent to a cardiac rehab and prevention program. When you hear *rehab,* you might picture a program offering addiction counselling in a secluded retreat. That's not what cardiac rehab is like. It's also quite different from rehabilitation for a debilitating stroke, where the goal is to help you regain vital function and motor skills. Cardiac rehab is a medically supervised program focusing on exercise, lifestyle modification and control of your risk factors through education. If you are living with heart disease and recovering from a heart attack or coronary heart procedure, you will improve your health and well-being by participating in a rehab program. Among other preventive measures, cardiac rehab offers lifestyle and dietary advice from medical professionals as well as guidance on how to control your cholesterol. One of the major components of rehab is to provide you with excellent information and encouragement to start an exercise and lifestyle plan. You can start small—by incorporating walking in your daily routine, along with making important dietary changes. It's short-term pain for long-term gain—a motto I live by.

❤ You need to know: If you are living with coronary heart disease, you should ask your doctor if you are on an anti-platelet therapy, an ACE inhibitor and cholesterol medication. You also need to ask whether or not your blood pressure is in the normal range—your doctor will determine what "normal"

means in your particular case—and whether it is appropriate for you to be on a drug such as a beta blocker. If you have not been referred to cardiac rehab after a heart attack, you should ask your doctor to do so.

In addition to the ABCs of treatment, you may be a candidate for invasive medical procedures and even major surgery. You may also be curious about any non-traditional and alternative treatments available to you. The next section discusses what you need to know about these topics.

Alternative Drugs and Treatments

It has amazed me over the years to find out that people will pay more for non-prescription medications and treatments than actual prescription drugs. Complementary and alternative medical therapy (or CAM), such as chelation therapy, herbal medications and acupuncture, is big business. Millions of dollars are spent every year on natural or alternative therapies for heart disease, without any rigorous evaluations of their use. As a physician, I'm trained in a traditional medical model, which means I want to see the evidence as to why a drug or treatment is effective. However, most complementary and alternative therapies have not been studied in a proper, scientific way. Unfortunately, many companies are promoting unproven treatments for profit, and patients are looking for that "magic bullet" to cure their problems. The reality is, lifestyle changes and evidence-based medications are the only scientifically endorsed ways to reduce your risk.

That said, I understand that many people have different opinions on this issue than I do—particularly those trained in non-traditional medicine. I've always encouraged my patients to tell me all the alternative or complementary therapies or medications they are undergoing or taking, as it's important for me to know about them. If my patients want to try non-traditional therapy, I ask them to do so in addition to, rather than instead of, the pills or treatments I prescribe. In other words, consider these treatments as *complementary* to the tried and true. I'm most concerned when patients embrace alternative therapies instead of taking their cholesterol or blood pressure pills or, even worse, instead of having recommended procedures such as angioplasty or bypass surgery.

In contrast, if CAM treatments are used as an *alternative* to traditional medicine, the disease of atherosclerosis can progress, and the results can be fatal. I have had a patient die after he refused bypass surgery and opted for chelation therapy. I have also had several patients opt for chelation therapy and come back to see me after it failed to work. The problem is that if your disease progresses, you may not be as good a candidate for bypass surgery down the road. Two of my patients were, at one point, candidates for bypass surgery. Both opted instead for chelation therapy. By the time they realized the chelation therapy was not working, their disease was so severe that they no longer qualified for a bypass.

❤ **You need to know: If you opt for complementary therapies, they should be taken in addition to traditional, evidence-based medications rather than as alternatives to proven treatments.**

Another belief system I have encountered over the years is "If it's natural, it's healthy." Let me explain why this is certainly not the case. The classic example is the cardiac medication digoxin, otherwise known as digitalis. Used for hundreds of years in treating heart rhythms and heart failure, digitalis is technically a "natural" product, extracted from the plant foxglove. But that doesn't necessarily make it "healthy." Digitalis needs to be controlled, regulated and prescribed based on evidence. Countless Canadians will remember a tragic series of deaths of pediatric heart patients in the 1980s at Toronto's SickKids hospital; the children were poisoned by overdoses of digoxin.

I remember clearly the case of a man who came in to the ER unconscious when I was a resident. He was found to have high digitalis levels in his blood—only he wasn't supposed to be on the medication. Although we never knew the truth, it seemed that he had been poisoned. Since doctors don't routinely screen for digitalis, it would have been invisible. Fortuitously, a junior intern had ordered the test by accident. The patient survived—but only by a happy accident!

Years later, I saw a patient who told me he was taking a natural "remedy" called hawthorn berries. When I looked up information on this natural product, I realized it was a weaker composition of a phosphodiesterase inhibitor, a medication used for some years in cardiology. This medication was tested in the regulated pill form in a clinical trial. As it turns out, it did have an effect on the heart and blood vessels—just not a beneficial one. In the clinical trial, more people taking the medication had side effects than those taking a placebo, or fake medication. This medication was taken off the market, but hawthorn berries are still available in various health food stores.

Complementary and alternative therapies can interfere with your prescription medications. Patients don't always tell their doctors about the non-prescription medication they are on. This can cause dangerous problems. If you are insisting on taking complementary and alternative therapies, at least tell your doctor what you're taking.

❤ **You need to know: If you are taking complementary or alternative therapies, you need to talk to your doctor about it. Some of these therapies can be dangerous or can interfere with your prescription medications.**

Interventions: Angioplasty, or PCI

In addition to medications for coronary artery disease, you may need an intervention—a surgical procedure—to open up narrowings or blockages in blood flow to your heart. This is usually the case right after a heart attack or if you are having frequent angina (chest discomfort). One of the commonly performed procedures in cardiology is called angioplasty, or percutaneous coronary intervention (PCI). Percutaneous means "through the skin." A coronary angioplasty, or PCI, is similar to an angiogram (see Chapter 6). However, in addition to squirting dye into your heart to take pictures, a wire with a balloon is attached to the catheter tube, which is then sent into your coronary artery. This small, non-inflated balloon is put through the narrowing seen on the angiogram. It's then inflated in order to open up the narrowing, thus improving blood flow.

The medical short form for this procedure is POBA, which stands for plain old balloon angioplasty. It's an effective intervention. However, because the balloon essentially disrupts the artery and smashes the cholesterol plaque against your blood vessel wall, a "reaction to injury" may occur inside the vessel. This is the body's attempt to heal after the vessel has been hurt. But it can cause problems. Cells grow within the vessel wall to try to heal the artery. The cells can grow inward or become thick in this area, which may lead to a renarrowing of the artery. This is called restenosis.

Here are some other terms you should know relating to angioplasty:

Stents: A stent is a metal strut that is placed in your artery during a balloon angioplasty. Its goal is to prevent a renarrowing of the blood vessel. In the old days, before stenting, close to 40% of angioplasties ended up with restenosis. Stents have cut restenosis rates in half.

Stenting an Artery

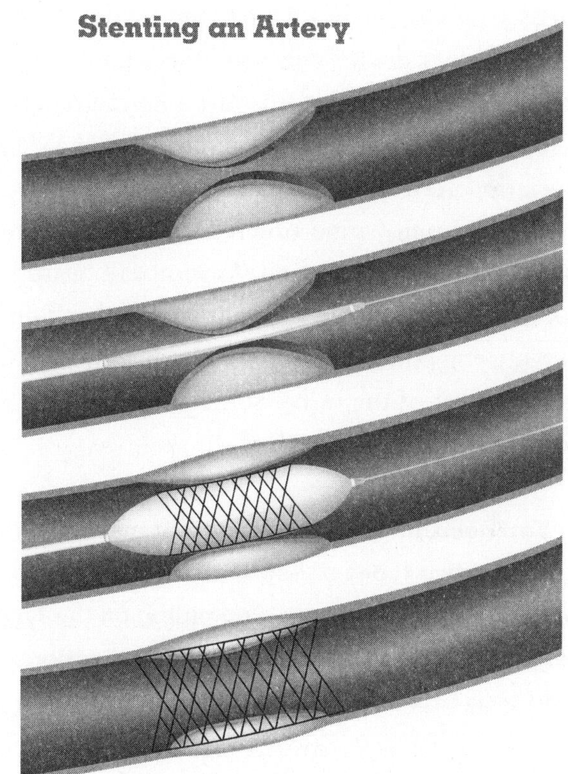

Your body heals after an angioplasty and stent insertion by growing a blood vessel lining around the metal strut. With time, the stent is incorporated into your artery. The growth of the lining can take up to two months or, with newer drug-eluting stents, approximately a year. Until the lining completely forms, the metal struts in the stent are "sticky," and you are at risk of a blood clot forming on the stent. This, of course, elevates your risk of heart attack. It's therefore crucial for you to take dual antiplatelet therapy—a combination of medications such as clopidogrel and ASA—after your angioplasty and stent insertion. If you find yourself bleeding or bruising after your stent insertion, you still need to continue with your ASA or Aspirin-like medications as well as your clopidogrel. Don't stop taking these medications—even if another doctor tells you otherwise. I'll give you a real-life example. One of my patients saw a dermatologist for a rash she had developed—a reaction to clopidogrel. Her dermatologist saw association between the drug and the rash and, in a decision that sends chills up my spine, ordered her to stop the medication. The results could have been fatal. As soon as I heard about it, thankfully only six days later, I got the patient back on track with her antiplatelet medication. I prescribed her another drug to prevent the side effect of the rash—something I could have done earlier had I known about the rash.

❤ **You need to know: After a stent insertion, you need to be on at least two types of Aspirin-like medications for anywhere from two months to a year, depending on the type of stent. You should never stop your antiplatelet medications without talking to your cardiologist—even if you are having side effects.**

Bare metal and drug-eluting stents: To complicate matters further, there are different types of stents. Bare metal came on the scene first; but they were not always effective in preventing renarrowing of the artery. As a consequence, a newer generation of stents has been developed in order to better prevent restenosis. These are drug-eluting stents (DES), which are coated with certain medications that prevent the blood vessel from growing inward and renarrowing. Unfortunately, this same medication also prevents the cells that line the artery (endothelial cells) from growing. As a consequence, if you are a patient who's had a drug-eluting stent inserted, part of your coronary artery may be very sticky to blood platelets. Again, it can take up to a year for your endothelial cells to grow and cover the inside of the stent—hence the need to be on antiplatelet medications. It can be fatal to stop taking antiplatelet medications prior to a year after a drug-eluting stent is inserted (depending on the particular type of drug-eluting stent you have). Many patients do well with drug-eluting stents, but if you have this particular kind of stent, talk with your doctor about the duration of your course of antiplatelet medication. As well as staying on this medication for as long as your doctor advises, you should continue taking cholesterol-lowering medications and other drugs as a matter of course to treat your heart disease.

> There's been no shortage of controversy in the last few years about the safety of drug-eluting stents and their links to patient deaths. But, in fact, research shows that the majority of patients who had heart attacks and died after stent therapy had stopped using the antiplatelet medication six months, rather than a year, after a stent's insertion. That's why it's important to stay on your medication for as long as your doctor advises.

When a patient is on a powerful antiplatelet agent, certain dilemmas may arise. Consider, for example, if the patient needs to have surgery for another medical issue and, as a result, has to stop taking her medication. One of my patients, the mother of a close friend, had arthritis and needed hip surgery. She also had had a heart attack and received a drug-eluting stent in her left anterior descending artery. If she proceeded with the hip surgery, she'd have to stop her antiplatelet medication. This was not an easy situation. Her hip was causing chronic pain and disability.

But the condition was not life threatening. I told my friend and her mother that if the scenario involved my mother, I would wait, even if that meant living with the pain of arthritis. In fact, this is what she did. After a year, her antiplatelet medications were stopped transiently, and she had successful hip surgery.

I faced another difficult situation with a young woman who had coronary heart disease. In one respect, she was a good candidate for angioplasty: She had a serious narrowing of blood flow in her left anterior descending artery. But she didn't actually need the angioplasty because evidence suggested she would do well taking medications alone. In this particular case, this young woman was doing well by taking anti-angina pills. She rock climbed and skied and had a high threshold for exercise. She had very few complaints except when she was exerting herself to an extreme. According to an extensive clinical trial, certain patients like her do just as well on cholesterol-lowering medications and ACE inhibitors as they would if they received an angioplasty. As a consequence, we elected not to proceed with angioplasty but rather to follow her carefully over time to make sure she did not get worse. In retrospect, this was the right decision. Four months after receiving her diagnosis of heart disease, she was found to have an ovarian tumour, which needed removal. Fortunately it was benign, but if we had decided to proceed with angioplasty, and she had needed drug-eluting stents, her surgery for her tumour may have had to have been delayed.

Major Surgery: Coronary Artery Bypass

The most common form of surgery for people with heart disease is coronary artery bypass graft (CABG) surgery. In this surgery, the physician is bypassing the narrowed vessels to the heart, using the body's natural blood vessels, usually veins or arteries taken from elsewhere in the body. A bypass is open-heart surgery that requires the patient to be on a heart–lung machine so that blood can be diverted to the brain while the surgeon operates on the heart. It's a safe procedure in the hands of a good surgeon. The risks of CABG surgery have decreased over the years with better surgical and anesthetic techniques. But make no mistake: It's a big operation. I tell my patients that for the first few months after bypass surgery, they will feel as if a truck ran them over. That's because, to get to the heart, the surgeon has to cut open the sternum, or breastbone, and pry open the ribs.

Coronary Artery Bypass Surgery

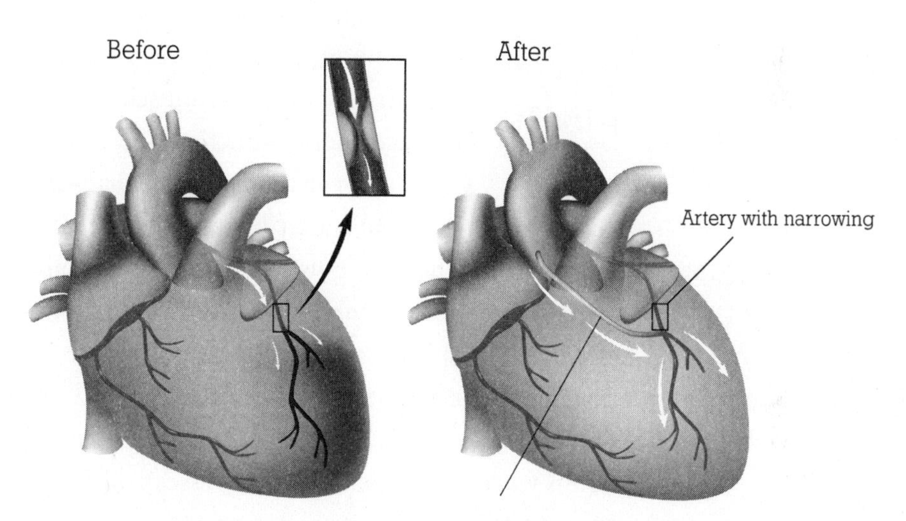

How is a bypass performed? With a bypass, an artery from your chest wall (for example, the left internal mammary artery) is attached to your aorta, the blood vessel from which your coronary arteries branch off. In addition to arteries, a surgeon will often use veins from the legs as bypass grafts. A bypass is created and sewn from the aorta to an area beyond the narrowing in your coronary arteries. The number of bypasses depends on the location of the narrowing. For example, you can have one narrowing in the left

There are two main coronary arteries that supply blood to your heart: the right and the left coronary artery. The left further branches into two: the circumflex coronary artery and the left anterior descending (LAD) artery. The former, the circumflex artery, runs deeper into your heart muscle. Instead of the circumflex, it's actually its branches—called the OM arteries—that are bypassed. Often, as well, bypasses will be put on branches of the anterior descending artery—the diagonal arteries.

main artery that supplies blood to most of your heart. But it will require several bypasses, or detours, so that blood can reach the branch arteries. Therefore one narrowing—say it's a narrowing of the left main artery—may require four bypasses; the left main supplies the left anterior descending artery, the diagonal artery, the circumflex artery and the obtuse marginal (OM) arteries. The risk of the surgery is usually not dependent on the number of bypasses but on the strength of your heart-muscle function; your age, kidney function and nutrition status; and whether you have diabetes.

Usually after bypass surgery, angina will improve because your heart is now receiving enough blood. But a more compelling reason that cardiologists recommend bypass surgery is that it allows patients—especially those with multi-vessel coronary artery disease and weakened heart muscles—to live longer. Feel better, live longer. Not a bad outcome!

It's a common worry for patients that bypasses will not last. In fact, when I went to medical school before cholesterol medications were routinely prescribed, only vein bypasses were used and not arterial bypasses. Vein bypasses remained effective only 50% of the time 10 years after the surgery. Arterial bypasses, however, have a 90% chance of remaining open 10 years down the road. Nowadays, modern medications and aggressive lifestyle modifications have improved the odds even more of keeping your bypasses healthy and open.

I can't stress enough the importance of taking ongoing medications after bypass surgery. This is especially so 5 or 10 years down the road, when your medical crisis starts feeling like part of a distant, hazy past. Frequently, I'll see a patient who hasn't visited a cardiologist or physician for up to a decade after bypass surgery and is no longer on any medication, not even simple ASA. Anyone who's had bypass surgery or angioplasty, and anyone who's been treated with medications for coronary heart disease, needs to be on ASA in addition to cholesterol-lowering medications—for life.

♥ You need to know: If you or a family member has had a bypass, you must take medications such as ASA and cholesterol-lowering drugs daily to prevent development of further disease in the bypasses.

Not everyone needs, or is a candidate for, bypass surgery. Sometimes, your coronary arteries will be damaged or shaped in such a way that a bypass is not possible to perform. It's like construction on a busy highway. If the road crew creates an effective detour, cars can keep flowing around the blockage and end up coasting along on a part of the highway beyond the construction. However, if the detour diverts the highway traffic to a bicycle path, there's no point. Likewise, patients don't make good candidates for coronary artery bypass surgery when their distal blood vessels are too small—in other words, the blood vessels beyond the major narrowing are too small to handle a detour, or bypass.

Who Gets Which Treatment?

Now you know all about the treatment options available in cardiac care. So which option is the right one for you? The answer is that all people with heart disease may have one of three treatments: medications alone, angioplasty (plus medications) or major surgery (plus medications). Deciding what's best for you or your loved one depends on several factors.

In general, if you haven't had a heart attack but you've been diagnosed with chronic coronary disease, you may do well on medications alone—unless you have frequent angina or your stress test or scan results are very abnormal, suggesting that your risk has increased.

If you have had a recent heart attack, you will likely go on to have an angiogram and then, where appropriate, have angioplasty or bypass surgery. Which one in particular? It's a complex decision. In most medical institutions, if a patient has had an angiogram and the nature of the narrowings doesn't immediately indicate the need for one procedure over another, the case is discussed with both cardiologists and cardiac surgeons before a course of action is offered. Regardless of the treatment chosen, you'll be on medications to control recurrence of the disease.

Many people think that having a high-tech procedure, whether it's surgery or angioplasty, is often the superior treatment for something as serious as chronic heart disease. But that's not always the case. I also have many patients who do not require such interventions. In general, the better your exercise tolerance on a treadmill test, the less debilitating your chest pain and the more normal your heart-muscle function is, the more likely you are to do well on medications alone. Obviously, this is an individual discussion between a patient and his cardiologist. Ask your doctor lots of probing questions!

❤ **You need to know: All patients with heart disease may have one of three treatments: medications, angioplasty (with medications) or surgery (with medications). Some patients with chronic coronary disease do well on medications alone. But if you have had a recent heart attack, you should likely have an angiogram and, where appropriate, angioplasty or surgery.**

Although its results are the subject of debate within the medical community, the COURAGE trial has changed how many cardiologists practise medicine. Because of this trial, doctors are now performing fewer angioplasties in favour of using medications alone to treat narrowed coronary arteries. COURAGE stands for Clinical Outcomes Utilizing Revascularization and Aggressive Drug Evaluation. The findings of the study were presented in 2007 at a conference in Louisiana and simultaneously published in the *New England Journal of Medicine*. The COURAGE trial was conducted on more than 2,200 patients with chronic stable coronary disease (but no recent heart attacks).[6] The patients all had angiograms, and they received one of two treatments: an angioplasty plus medications or medications alone. The study showed that both treatments, in effect, worked: There was no difference in survival or recurrent chance of heart attack between the patients over time. All of the study's patients were also on aggressive preventive medications—focused on lowering cholesterol and blood pressure—and made significant lifestyle changes.

Treating a Heart Attack

I want to end this chapter with heart attacks—mainly to emphasize the life-saving nature of early response in treating them. If you have a heart attack, your treatment greatly depends on how quickly you get to the hospital. Urge your family and friends to be equipped with an emergency plan. The Heart and Stroke Foundation urges us all to respond by dialling 9-1-1 or the local emergency number and to be prepared by being trained to administer cardiopulmonary resuscitation (CPR) if someone collapses and appears unresponsive. According to the Foundation, only 40% of all Canadians trained in CPR know what to do to resuscitate a person who's had a heart attack.[7] The appropriate course of action is this: Don't delay, call an ambulance. Don't worry about the usual protocol of "looking, listening and feeling" for a pulse or signs of breathing. If you know CPR—and more of us should learn the procedure—focus on pushing "fast and hard." For more details, consult the Heart and Stroke Foundation's guidelines at www.heartandstroke.ca/CPRguidelines.

If you have a heart attack, time is crucial. Acute heart attacks are not something you and your doctor want to address days or weeks after they happen. Medical interventions must be performed in an emergency framework. In a sense, then, anyone who suffers a heart attack is, to some degree, the architect of her destiny—the key to getting good care is immediate recognition of the symptoms.

A heart attack occurs when junk in the arteries (atherosclerosis) becomes unstable and tries to grow. The piece of unstable junk, or plaque, attracts platelets, leading to a blood clot. If the blood clot has not fully formed, then the type of heart attack is usually what we consider less severe. In contrast, when a full blood clot disrupts flow to the coronary artery, the heart attack is more severe, and the treatment is to open up the blood clot. That can occur through either clot-busting medication such as thrombolytics or by going straight to the catheterization lab and receiving angioplasty.

Angioplasty is an effective way of restoring blood flow to the artery and can even be used during an acute heart attack if you have a blood clot in the artery—as long as you get to the cath lab in time. Angioplasty that's done around the time of a heart attack is called primary angioplasty, as it is the primary treatment for the attack.

Still, you won't know what type of heart attack you are having until you get to the hospital! The single most important thing to do is get to the hospital fast. It's that simple. If you have signs or symptoms that suggest a heart attack, call 9-1-1 without delay.

Clot-busting medications will help if your heart attack is severe (called ST elevation MI) but you can't get to a cardiac catheterization lab quickly. Say, for example, you live in a remote area, and the nearest hospital does not have a cath lab. You will be prescribed clot-busting medication to get rid of the clot blocking your arteries. One such drug is called tissue plasminogen activator (TPA). Sometimes patients are transferred from one hospital to another to receive an angioplasty. But studies show that receiving clot-busting agents is almost as good as, if not better than, having an angioplasty performed too late.

If you're having a heart attack that's less severe (called non-ST MI), you may receive intravenous or injectable blood thinners such as heparin (as a side note, some injectable types of heparin are not appropriate for people who have kidney disease). Once you have been given blood thinners for 48 hours, if the pain has settled down, but if your ECG and blood tests show abnormalities, you may go on to an angiogram and a possible angioplasty. You may also be made to do a treadmill stress test to evaluate how your heart functions on exertion. If you have an abnormal treadmill test or a nuclear perfusion (blood flow) scan after a heart attack, your doctor may order an angiogram—because your risk of future problems is increased. Some patients, however, do not need angiograms after heart attacks because their risk can be managed by medications alone.

If you or a family member has been discharged from hospital after a heart attack and did not receive an angiogram, ask the doctor to explain why. A cardiac specialist should be able to explain the reasons thoroughly.

❤ **You need to know: If you or a family member were discharged from hospital after a heart attack without receiving an angiogram, you should ask: "Why wasn't an angiogram performed?" A cardiac specialist will be able to take you through the answer.**

I would be remiss if I didn't dispel the myths related to treatment of a heart attack. You may have seen or received dangerous emails from well-meaning friends that claim to have important tips about the signs and symptoms of a heart attack or stroke. Over the years, I have seen these emails, usually sent on by my mother or her friends, asking, "Is this really true?"

There are some crazy ones out there. Some "tips" include sitting in unusual positions, hiccupping and deep breathing while having a heart attack. Press delete immediately! Having a heart attack or stroke is a very serious event that requires immediate medical attention. If you want to use the Internet to gain some helpful information on signs and symptoms, visit the Heart and Stroke Foundation's site at www.heartandstroke.ca/heartsigns. Also, check out my lists of dos and don'ts if you or a loved one is experiencing signs of a heart attack.

My "Do" List

DO call 9-1-1 or your local emergency number immediately or have someone call for you.

DO keep an emergency list of numbers of family and friends near the phone at all times; the paramedics may need to contact people on your behalf.

DO stop all activity and sit or lie down, in whatever position is most comfortable. If you are driving, pull to the side of the road and stop your car.

DO take a normal dosage of nitroglycerine if you're on the medication. If you are experiencing chest pain and are not already on ASA, chew and swallow one adult 325 mg tablet or two 81 mg (low dose) ASA. Note that acetaminophen (commonly known as Tylenol) and ibuprofen (Advil) do not work in the same way as ASA. Only ASA will help in an emergency situation.

My "Don't" List

DON'T ignore your signs and symptoms and take your son to a soccer practice instead of taking yourself to the emergency room.

DON'T tell yourself this is indigestion and pick up your mother from her seniors class.
DON'T debate with your spouse whether or not this could be your heart and decide to take a Tums and go to bed instead.
DON'T email your doctor that you are having chest pain—and wait for him to respond.
DON'T decide to get on a plane home from Florida and have your doctor check it out in a day or so, even if you do not have health insurance while on holiday.
DON'T make an appointment with your family doctor a week later because you have an important work presentation the following day.

These tips may sound ridiculous, but I base them all on true events. Even the smartest people will often be in denial. Knowing what to do and actually doing it are two different things!

Time and time again, I meet men and women who have tried to put off dealing with their heart disease. It's akin to adopting an "out of sight, out of mind" mentality. The less they think about their heart health, the more they believe their issues will go away. Of course, that's always a dangerous approach.

One of my patients is a 57-year-old mother of grown children who has a career as a registered nurse. At work and at home, she attended to the needs of everyone around her. But despite her medical background, she remained in denial about her own health. She has lived with type 1 diabetes for many years. She had high blood pressure and recurrent angina (the chest pain that results from coronary heart disease). Living with angina had greatly limited her activity, and yet she took on a lot of night shifts at the hospital where she works and never really slowed down or addressed her risk factors. She was simply not making her health a priority. It's a common pattern: She had gone through several episodes in her younger years when she didn't watch her blood sugars. She did not take her own health as seriously as caring for her children or her patients. From time to time, she went off her diabetic medication. Sometimes, she'd have an "aha moment" and begin to take the right steps in caring for her health, but it wouldn't take long before she reverted back to her old habits. At a certain point in time, she also arbitrarily decided to stop her cholesterol medication. When you have diabetes, as she did, cholesterol is essential to control. This was the final straw for her body. After experiencing more and more chest pain, she had a heart attack. By the time I met her, after her heart attack, she was full of regret. Sadly, however, she couldn't undo the damage that was done. Unfortunately, like most people, she had to experience a major health crisis to start heeding the medical advice that was offered her years before.

It's my hope that if you're reading this book, you will have plenty of reason not to let the same thing happen to you. When it comes to your health, don't wait for something terrible to happen before taking action. Arm yourself with the information in this book, engage in a dialogue with your doctor, take care of yourself, take your medications and don't ignore your symptoms—take charge instead!

11

TREATMENTS FOR ARRHYTHMIAS

"My 21-year-old daughter went to hospital with a fast heart rate. The doctors say she can have an ablation. What does this involve?"

In this case, the young woman was experiencing extra heartbeats—causing symptoms that her doctor felt warranted an ablation. An ablation is an invasive surgical procedure where the short-circuit that causes the abnormal heartbeat is corrected. In fact, *ablating* means getting rid of the short-circuit in the heart by either burning or freezing it. We'll get to the reasons a patient would require an ablation later in this chapter. But first, let's recap the basics of arrhythmias. Rhythm disturbances of the heart—otherwise known as arrhythmias—are common conditions. Arrhythmias range in severity and can result from either fast or slow heartbeats. They appear at all stages of life, but non-serious arrhythmias are often seen in younger, healthier adults. Some palpitations are benign, meaning you don't have to worry about them. At the other end of the spectrum, some arrhythmias can be life threatening.

Benign Palpitations

As a rule, if you are otherwise healthy, do not have heart-muscle damage and are not fainting from extra beats, the palpitations are harmless and there's no need for treatment. All the same, experiencing palpitations can be vexing. In fact, when I see patients who have a benign arrhythmia, I ask if they are bothered by it, worried by it—or both. Patients who are bothered by palpitations may benefit from medications that will reduce the tendency for extra beats. These drugs are usually beta blockers or calcium channel blockers. Beta blockers block the adrenalin to the heart and slow your pulse. Calcium channel blockers are heart drugs that can also slow the impulses in your heart. These drugs are usually well tolerated. They're not considered anti-arrhythmic drugs, which have the potential for more serious side effects. That said, I usually don't prescribe medications after a patient's initial assessment for benign palpitations. My immediate task is to reassure you that there is nothing to worry about and, then, to wait to see the impact of this news on the "bother factor." If three to six months later, you are still having significant symptoms, we'll consider medication.

In contrast to benign palpitations, if you are fainting because of arrhythmias, then you will need to be treated. Which form of treatment you receive depends on whether your heart is beating too slowly (called bradycardia) or too quickly (tachycardia). Let's discuss one at a time.

Slow Beats and Heart Block

If you have slow heartbeats, electrical signals from the top part of your heart (the atria) are blocked before they reach the bottom part of your heart (the ventricles). If your doctor tells you that you have a "heart block," it means the electrical impulses that normally travel from the top part of your heart into the ventricles are slowed down or blocked somewhere along the way. Sometimes, this slowing down is not serious whatsoever. For instance, if your doctor sees an electrocardiogram result that shows first-degree heart block, this means the electricity is simply taking time to go through the atrium to the ventricle. First-degree heart block is not serious at all.

Second-degree heart block comes in two forms. One is called type 1 (or Wenckebach). This is a variation on normal experienced by healthy people. With Wenckebach, your heart slows down temporarily; it can occur to many of us when we sleep. On the other hand, there's type 2 second-degree AV block. It's a serious problem with the electrical system in the heart and may be a warning sign that electrical impulses are not getting through as they normally should. If you are light-headed or having fainting episodes with this form of heart block, you may benefit from a pacemaker. A pacemaker is a small device inserted under the skin in your upper chest when there is serious heart block; its wire leads attach into the heart and create electrical impulses. In other words, a pacemaker creates heartbeats for you.

Third-degree, or complete, heart block essentially means the atrium is not "talking to" the ventricles electrically. Usually, if you have complete heart block, you will experience light-headedness or fainting. If that is the case, then your doctor will advise that a pacemaker be inserted in your body. It's more common for elderly patients to experience these slow arrhythmias, which require pacemakers, rather than younger patients.

Pacemakers are very sophisticated devices. They can sense what is happening in your heart. If your heart's natural electrical system is working well, they usually stop pacing, or go into standby. Pacemakers come out to work only when your heart needs it. Inserting a pacemaker is a relatively minor procedure; it's much smaller surgery than open-heart surgery.

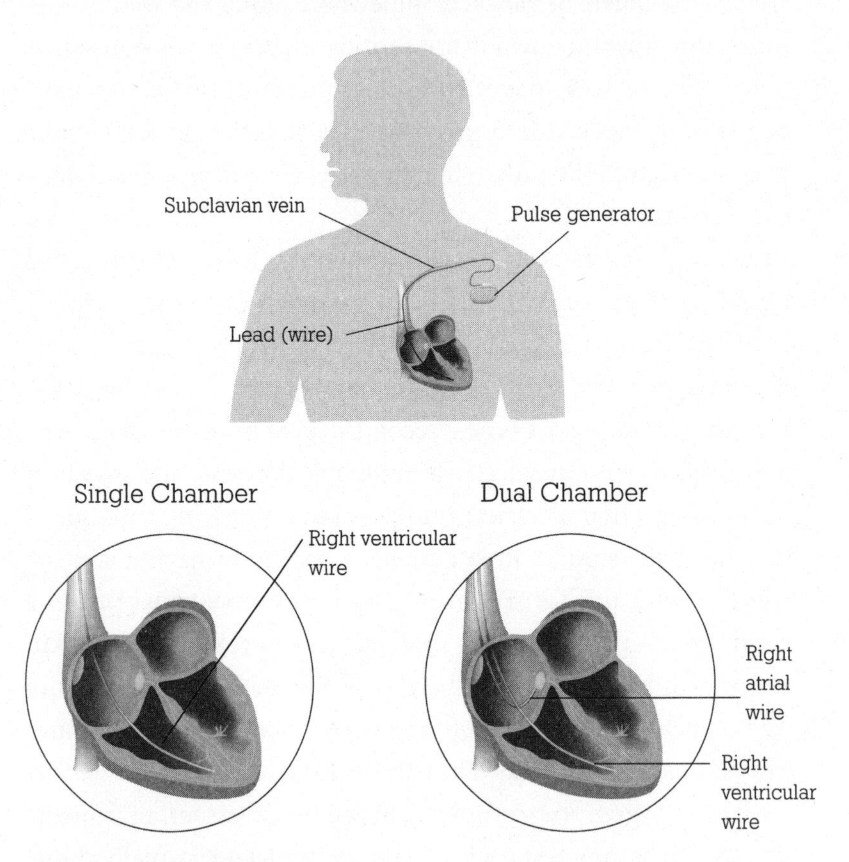

Fast Heart Rhythms: Supraventricular Tachycardia (SVT)

As we learned earlier, SVT is the general term for a group of disorders in which fast or extra beats originate from the top part of the heart (the atria). Most SVT disorders are non-serious, with the exception of atrial fibrillation and atrial flutter (described next).

The treatment of SVT depends on the type of disorder and severity of symptoms. Certain types of SVT noticeably come on and go away quickly. Many patients who have the most common type of SVT—a short-circuit called AVNRT—experience rapid heart action that may make them, on occasion, feel mildly unwell or short of breath. However, these episodes may be brief or infrequent. In these cases, often no therapy is required. At the other end of the spectrum, there are patients who are quite symptomatic. They routinely either pass out, feel unwell or are lightheaded because of SVT. If your doctor advises specific treatment for SVT, it would take the form of either an ablation procedure, which involves using a catheter to correct the short-circuit, or medications to slow the impulse in the short-circuit.

I have a patient with SVT who is 63 years old and retired. He is an active man and avid cycler who has followed a heart-healthy lifestyle since he quit smoking a decade ago. Over the last few years, however, he has experienced high blood pressure. He described having his first experience with symptoms of arrhythmia when he was relaxing at home, reading a book and listening to classical music. Suddenly, he felt an onset of rapid heart action—his heart was racing, and it didn't stop for several hours. He did not lose consciousness during this episode, but every 10 days or so, the palpitations would return. I asked him to wear a loop monitor (see Chapter 7) in order to assess the arrhythmia over a period of time. Ultimately, this patient was feeling weak because of his symptoms as well as experiencing hemodynamic compromise—meaning his brain wasn't getting enough blood because his heart was beating too fast to be effective. Because his quality of life was greatly affected by his SVT, he was a good candidate for an ablation. He had the procedure and has been doing well ever since without any recurrent symptoms.

Unlike this patient, you may experience infrequent SVT symptoms. A common approach in this case is the "pill in the pocket" technique. In other words, you don't need to be on medications for years at a time to prevent only sporadic episodes of SVT. Instead, you can take a medication such as a beta blocker, a calcium channel blocker or even an anti-arrhythmic drug as soon as you feel the onset of fast heartbeats to try to "break" the arrhythmia. Since many of the common SVTs are related to short-circuits occurring through the AV node of your heart, anything that can slow down or break a short-circuit in the node, medication or otherwise, is useful. Sometimes simple manoeuvres you can do on your own will do the trick. As we covered in Chapter 5, the vagus nerve is the stop-sign nerve in your body—it slows the heart rate down. The vagus nerve can also affect the AV node. You can increase the vagus nerve's activity by bearing down, as if you are about to have a bowel movement, or hyperventilating into a paper bag.

Atrial Fibrillation

If you are diagnosed with this potentially serious condition, your heart is beating in an irregular and disorganized manner. Atrial fibrillation, or A-fib, may be associated with a variety of issues (see Chapter 9), including sleep apnea and disease of the mitral valve. It's also associated with hypertension (high blood pressure), which creates increased pressure in the left ventricle of the heart and, in turn, can lead to pressure that causes your heart's left atrium to stretch. An enlarged left atrium increases the chances that you may develop an irregular heartbeat. You can experience significant consequences of atrial fibrillation. Chief among them is an increased risk of having a stroke. With atrial fibrillation, a blood clot can form in the top part of your heart when the atrium is fibrillating, or beating irregularly. This clot can break off from within the heart and travel up through the aorta to the blood vessels in the brain. This blood clot can disrupt blood flow to your brain, causing a brain attack, or stroke.

♥ You need to know: If you or a family member has atrial fibrillation, the greatest health concern is a risk of stroke. Talk to your doctor to see if you are at risk and whether you need to be put on a blood thinner.

To prevent the clots from forming, many patients with atrial fibrillation must take a blood thinner, the most common of which is warfarin (or Coumadin). Believe it or not, this medication was originally used as a rat poison, but today warfarin is both a safe and effective drug. If you are on warfarin, you will have to go for regular blood work to monitor the drug's efficacy. The amount of warfarin required varies from patient to patient. For the medication to work, it has to thin the blood within a very narrow range of effectiveness. The blood test tells your doctor how well the drug is working. If your blood is not thin enough on warfarin, your risk of stroke and clotting will not be reduced, and if your blood is *too* thin, you are at risk of experiencing bleeding. Warfarin also has various food and drug interactions, so it's important that you talk to your pharmacist and physician to review the drug closely.

❤ **You need to know: If you are on warfarin for atrial fibrillation, then it's crucial to undergo regular blood tests to monitor the drug's effectiveness.**

One of my patients is a 46-year-old who is struggling with a weight problem and has high blood pressure and high cholesterol. His symptoms began with shortness of breath, which eventually turned out not to be related to coronary heart disease but to arrhythmia. At one point, he experienced a sudden loss of vision and rushed to the emergency room. He had had a transient ischemic attack (or TIA). That's when the blood flow to the brain is disrupted for a brief period of time. We call it a "warning stroke." He was diagnosed with atrial fibrillation and has been on blood thinners ever since. However, I decided he was not a good candidate for warfarin. He's a pleasant guy, but he does not like to see doctors and could forget to have his warfarin blood test. We switched to a newer drug that protects him from the risk of stroke but doesn't require monitoring. In recent years, such newer blood thinners have appeared on the market that don't require you to take blood tests. These drugs have been proven effective in large studies. Unlike warfarin, however, some of the newer medications need to be taken more frequently—twice a day as opposed to once. Since using this medication, and making an effort to lose weight and change his lifestyle, my patient is at a much lower risk of having a future stroke.

It's important if you are taking these (or any other) medications to know the name of the drugs you're on. You also need to tell your family members precisely which medications you're taking. Carry the information on a card that is in your wallet at all times. In case of accidents and emergencies, doctors must know of any drugs that might cause you risk in surgery. Blood thinners, in particular, lead to a higher risk of bleeding. There's no blood test that allows doctors to identify the newer blood thinners, so you have to be able to tell your doctors what you've been taking.

Warfarin is monitored by a blood test called an international normalized ratio, or INR, which measures the clotting of the blood. In patients with atrial fibrillation and no other heart valve issues, we aim for an INR result of 2 to 3. If the INR is less than 2, your blood is not thin enough and your stroke risk is high. If the INR is over 3, your bleeding risk is slightly higher. There are subtleties here: I tell my patients that an INR of 1.8 is not acceptable but 3.1 or so may be. When I start my patients on warfarin, I will often order an INR once a week initially, and then, if stable, twice a month and then monthly. If you have been on warfarin and have never had an INR out of the 2 to 3 range, then a blood test every few months may be adequate. It is *not* okay, however, to be put on warfarin without having your blood checked regularly.

Studies show that if you are over the age of 65, especially if you are a woman, taking blood thinners is more useful for reducing the likelihood of a stroke than taking ASA. However, if you're very frail, fall often and are at risk of serious bleeding should you fall, then blood thinners may not be the right choice. Also, if you have atrial fibrillation and are otherwise healthy and under the age of 50, your condition is called "lone" atrial fibrillation. Instead of taking warfarin, these younger patients will do fine with 325 mg of ASA each day to reduce their risk of stroke. Some young, healthy patients do not even need ASA. Speak to your doctor to discuss which treatment is best for you.

On the other hand, you *must* be on an anticoagulation drug—either warfarin or a newer drug that doesn't require monitoring—if you've had a previous mini (TIA) or full stroke. You also need to be treated if you have valvular heart disease (a result of rheumatic fever, for instance) or if you are older and have high blood pressure, diabetes or congestive heart failure associated with your atrial fibrillation. As always, discuss the options with your doctor.

I have to add here that, despite all the advances in medical science, the treatment of patients with atrial fibrillation is a huge problem, with ongoing gaps in care. Recent studies suggest that only 10% of stroke patients who have been put on a drug such as warfarin fall into the therapeutic range—or the range where the drug is actually working. The other 90% of patients may be on warfarin, but their blood is not thinned enough. One-third of all stroke patients with atrial fibrillation are *not* put on any blood thinners but should be.[1]

In addition to stroke risk, atrial fibrillation can affect your quality of life. If you experience shortness of breath or fatigue or feel that your heart is racing, you may need medications such as beta blockers and calcium channel blockers to slow your heart rate down so you can feel better. If you experience severe limitations because of atrial fibrillation—meaning you have more aggravated symptoms—you may require more potent medications. These are anti-arrhythmic drugs (such as amiodarone, for example) to control the rhythm of the heart. Whether you take these drugs to slow the heart down (known as rate control) or to keep the heart in a normal rhythm (rhythm control), you will still need to be on blood thinners to lower the risk of stroke.

If your quality of life is severely impacted because of atrial fibrillation, and the medications are not proving effective, then you may also be a candidate for an ablation. An atrial fibrillation ablation is a procedure where the short-circuit that causes an irregular heart beat is corrected by burning or freezing areas within the atrium. This can be a complicated and lengthy procedure. As a result, ablations aren't recommended for most patients with atrial fibrillation. However, ablations are more commonly used if you have a slightly different rhythm problem—a "cousin" of atrial fibrillation called atrial flutter. Ablations for atrial flutter are usually very successful and are easier to perform.

Atrial Flutter

As with atrial fibrillation, atrial flutter is a serious irregularity of the heart that puts certain patients at risk for stroke. The risk of stroke with atrial flutter is the same as with atrial fibrillation. The difference is that atrial flutter, an irregular heartbeat at the top part of the heart, is more organized in its beating. As such, this short-circuit can be treated with an ablation, a procedure that is commonly performed in specialized cardiac centres. Not all patients with atrial flutter require an ablation. For instance, you may not need the procedure if you are completely asymptomatic—that is, you don't have any symptoms. Sometimes, if you have atrial flutter along with hypertension, medications for lowering your blood pressure may prove effective at controlling how fast your heart is beating. In any case, as with atrial fibrillation, you need to be on blood thinners if you are diagnosed with atrial flutter.

Cardioversion

If you have either atrial fibrillation or flutter, your doctor will decide either to slow your heart rate down (rate control) or try to keep your heart in a more normal rhythm (rhythm control). Changing the rhythm of your heart from abnormal to normal is called cardioversion. This can be done either with medication (chemical cardioversion) or with electricity (electrical cardioversion).

To maintain a normal rhythm, your doctor may prescribe medications called anti-arrhythmic drugs to you. Many anti-arrhythmic drugs are safe and useful, but they may also have pro-arrhythmic side effects—meaning they can put you at a slight risk of developing another rhythm problem. The alternative is to bring your heart into a normal rhythm with electricity. If you have a serious arrhythmia that causes your blood pressure to fall, you receive an electrical cardioversion in an emergency situation. If you have a chronic arrhythmia, you may opt for an elective electrical cardioversion.

Although it sounds scary, electrical cardioversion is actually safer overall than being put on multiple rhythm medications. Whether you need an electrical cardioversion depends on a range of issues regarding your condition and is a matter to discuss with your physicians. If your cardiologist recommends an electrical cardioversion, you should know that it's an effective and commonly performed day procedure. You'll come to the hospital, having had nothing to eat or drink after midnight, and be given a mild form of sedation (not a powerful anesthetic). You'll get an electrical charge through the chest wall and across your heart. This electricity will hopefully shock your heart back into a normal rhythm.

❤ **You need to know: Electrical cardioversion is a safe and effective procedure. It's used for many patients with atrial fibrillation or flutter who need to be in a normal rhythm, usually because of severe symptoms.**

Ventricular Tachycardia

As discussed in Chapter 9, a ventricular tachycardia (VT) is a fast heartbeat coming from the bottom part of your heart, or ventricles. If your doctor finds that you have VT, it needs to be evaluated by a cardiologist.

Sometimes VT is not serious: If your heart is otherwise normal, then it may be able to tolerate these fast, extra beats. I see patients who have ventricular tachycardia with otherwise structurally normal hearts, and they are not having symptoms. In these cases, little treatment is warranted, and sometimes patients may just need beta blockers.

Usually, however, ventricular tachycardia is more concerning. If your heart beats very quickly, it may not be able to work efficiently and allow blood to pump to the rest of your body—causing you to pass out. You are also at risk of having a cardiac arrest, meaning your heart can stop as a result of the fast heart rhythm. When this occurs, emergency measures such as a shock from an external defibrillator or internal defibrillator (see page 231) will often be life-saving.

If you have a weakened heart muscle, ventricular tachycardia can be a warning sign that there is danger ahead—even if you feel generally well. You may still benefit from an implanted defibrillator since you will be at great risk for sudden death because of the arrhythmia.

Ventricular Fibrillation

Ventricular fibrillation is one of the most serious arrhythmias you can have. It is characterized by a disorganized, fast rhythm coming from the bottom part of your heart. Since it's associated with a lack of blood flow, ventricular fibrillation is also a common cause of cardiac arrest (heart stop) during a heart attack. The treatment for ventricular fibrillation is to shock you out of this rhythm. This is one of the reasons we have defibrillators in busy places such as airports. A defibrillator can save your life if you have ventricular fibrillation.

Implantable Defibrillators

Implantable defibrillators have the ability to pace the heart when it is too slow or to shock the heart out of a fast rhythm. These small life-saving devices are implanted under the skin and attached to wire leads extending into the veins in your heart. A defibrillator looks like a pacemaker; however, it is more like a smart computer with a battery attached. Defibrillators can allow for electricity to go through the wires leading into the heart; the electricity can shock your heart out of a serious rhythm disturbance. Defibrillators also have pacemaker abilities, which means they can also speed up your heart if it's too slow.

Sometimes, defibrillators can overcome a fast rhythm of the heart without using a shock. This process is called overdrive pacing. Rather than shocking your heart, the pacemaker will go very fast—into overdrive—so the heart can go back into its normal rhythm. In fact, most defibrillators will go into overdrive pacing before they shock the heart in order to minimize a patient's pain. A shock can be painful, even if not harmful.

Usually defibrillators are implanted in people who have survived a cardiac arrest (when the heart stops) and are at risk for future cardiac arrests or in people who have had an extensive heart attack that has weakened the heart muscle. You'll remember from the start of the book that heart-muscle function is described by the term *ejection fraction*, or the percentage of blood ejected forward with every heartbeat.

In general, implantable defibrillators are useful if you have an ejection fraction of less than 30% and if you've had a heart attack in the past. People with an ejection fraction of less than 30% are at greatest risk of cardiac arrhythmia, even years after the heart attack.

Implantable defibrillators are not recommended if you have severe congestive heart failure (see Chapter 12) or have had a recent heart attack. Doctors also don't implant defibrillators in patients who are sick for other reasons. You need to allow a few months after your heart attack for your health to stabilize and for your medication to take effect. If you or a family member has had an extensive heart attack and has been left with heart-muscle damage, even if it was many years ago, ask your cardiologist whether you are a candidate for an implantable defibrillator.

As always, it's vital to engage in conversations with your doctor about how best to treat your arrhythmia. Explore the options available to you, and take all the therapies your cardiologist recommends seriously. If you have rhythm disturbances, in some cases you will need medications and treatments that have the ability to save your life and prevent the worst from happening. In other instances, you may need to reduce the symptoms of palpitations in order to improve your quality of life. In any circumstance, modern medicine can help you. Advances in the field are occurring all the time.

12

TREATMENT OF HEART FAILURE

"I was diagnosed with congestive heart failure, which sounds so final and hopeless. Is it really in my hands to control?"

Congestive heart failure (CHF or, simply, HF) is a serious condition affecting millions of people all over the world—so if you have it, you're not alone. CHF poses pressing dangers if left unmanaged, but the good news is, the disease can be treated by adopting heart-healthy lifestyle changes, in addition to taking important medications your cardiologist will prescribe.

A common cause of CHF occurs after a heart attack. After a heart attack, the dead heart muscle will not usually regain function. This places additional stress on the remaining, normally functioning heart muscle, which causes the heart to weaken further. However, certain medications can relieve this stress and prevent the heart from being "remodelled," or progressively enlarged.

Over the next few pages, we'll look at the range of treatment options available to you or your family members with CHF. For more information, I hasten to recommend the Heart and Stroke Foundation's excellent guide called *Managing Congestive Heart Failure*—which you can download from the website www.heartandstroke.ca.

Let's start by reviewing the types of CHF diagnoses. When your heart muscle is weakened, it's called systolic heart failure. Most often, your heart muscle is weakened as a result of a heart attack. It's less common, but heart failure may also be attributed to conditions such as diabetes, high blood pressure, excessive use of alcohol or drugs, or damaged or malfunctioning heart valves. Regardless of the cause, if the heart muscle is weakened, the management of the disease is generally the same. Treatment includes taking appropriate medications—including diuretics, ACE inhibitors and beta blockers—plus restricting salt and water intake. Your doctor may also determine if you are a candidate for high-tech therapies such as cardiac resynchronization (see page 238), an implantable defibrillator or even a heart transplant. If you have coronary artery disease in addition to heart failure, treating the coronary disease with angioplasty or bypass surgery may also be needed.

When the heart is stiff, rather than weak, the term is diastolic heart failure. This serious condition is often associated with high blood pressure. We know that patients who develop diastolic heart failure are at risk of recurrent hospitalization and even death, and they need to pay careful attention to their weight, their salt and water intake and their blood pressure.[1] According to various studies, it's less clear how specific drugs such as ACE inhibitors or beta blockers improve the outlook of diastolic heart failure.

Controlling Your Sodium

Watching your salt intake and keeping track of your weight is essential if you have been diagnosed with heart failure. Most women know that if they retain salt and water at a certain time of the month, their weight will go up on the scale. The same concept holds true if you have heart failure, during which your body tries to retain salt and water. Weight gain is one of the first signs of heart failure, and you will notice it before you see any swelling or have a buildup of fluid on your lungs, causing difficulty breathing. I tell my patients to be aware of the warning signs: If your weight goes up by 3 pounds (1.5 kg) in two days, it's unlikely due to your intake of fat or calories. It's more reasonable to assume the culprits are salt and water retention.

❤ **You need to know: The treatment of heart failure consists of making important lifestyle changes in addition to taking medications for the disease. If you have congestive heart failure, watching the salt in your diet and keeping track of your weight are critical.**

Salty food can, in some ways, push your heart over the edge. If you have a weakened heart muscle but are not experiencing heart failure, then your heart is somehow compensating for its weakened state. On the other hand, eating salt can cause you to decompensate and go into failure.

Along with throwing out the salt shaker at home (or hiding it from plain view), you have to restrain any penchant you have for processed foods that are high in salt, such as luncheon meats and canned and pickled foods. I recall a patient I saw several years ago who was admitted to hospital with heart failure. We couldn't find the cause of his condition—until we took a thorough history. It turns out that his wife, who had been preparing his meals, had departed for a month to visit her sister out of town. Instead of preparing meals on his own, my patient decided to order takeout at least twice a week. His meal choices—pizza, Chinese food and barbecued chicken—all contained a lot of salt, so much so that he gradually went into heart failure.

Most people don't pause to think about it, but fast-food restaurants, by and large, serve foods that have more salt than you can imagine. Yes, that means fries and burgers, but many other things we consume also have a staggering amount of sodium. For example, a serving of soda pop, even if it's diet, can have between 30 and 100 mg of sodium. That's high, especially if you have a daily limit. Barbecued chicken and barbecue sauce often have off-the-charts sodium content. The usual recommendation is that salt intake for anyone living with heart disease be less than 1,500 mg per day—if you have heart failure, it should be even lower. Most Canadians consume 3,400 mg of salt a day.

In addition to restricting salt and watching your weight, if you have heart failure you should adhere to a high-fibre diet because the water pills you are on can be constipating.

Vital Medications

Patients with heart failure may be on one or all of the following medications: diuretics (water pills), beta blockers and either angiotensin-converting enzyme (or ACE) inhibitors or angiotensin II receptor blockers (ARBs), in addition to digoxin. You should periodically review which of these medications you should take, and at what doses, with your family doctor. The prescription your doctor gives you will depend on a number of factors that may change over time—for instance, if your weight fluctuates, your prescription may have to be adjusted.

Diuretics are pills that help you combat fluid retention; these include a drug called furosemide, otherwise known as Lasix. Beta blockers block the flow of adrenalin to the heart and slow your pulse; blocking the adrenalin helps your heart muscle heal. ACE inhibitors curtail the production of a substance in the body that can raise your blood pressure and help the heart "remodel." ARBs have similar benefits for your blood pressure and are recommended as an alternative if you can't tolerate ACE inhibitors. (Some people develop a dry, hacking cough on ACE inhibitors.) Digoxin is also known as digitalis. It's shown to be able to strengthen the heart muscle slightly and keeps some patients with heart failure out of hospital.

❤ **You need to know: Medications for heart failure, which include diuretics, ACE inhibitors and beta blockers, can make you live longer in addition to making you feel better. If you have heart failure, never let a prescription run out. You should never change or stop your medication without notifying your physician.**

It's worthwhile to note that some groups of medications—usually arthritis or anti-inflammatory drugs—can cause salt and water retention and are usually not to be used by patients with congestive heart failure. If you are living with congestive heart failure, do not allow anyone to prescribe you an arthritis medication without checking with your heart specialist.

I use the term *specialist* because although congestive heart failure is a common problem, and can be well managed with the primary care of a family doctor, it's a complex disease that requires evaluation by an experienced cardiologist. There are even specific heart failure clinics cropping up throughout North America. Many patients take advantage of these clinics, which are staffed by specialists. Statistics show that patients who make regular visits to a specialized heart failure clinic generally feel better, live longer and

> If you develop heart failure with atrial fibrillation (an irregular heart beat), you will require drugs or electricity to enable your heart muscle to contract more effectively. Atrial fibrillation is a common cause of heart failure. If you have a weak, stiff or thickened heart muscle, up to 40% of the pumping action of the heart muscle (otherwise known as cardiac output) is a result of the top part of your heart (atria) contracting normally. However, in atrial fibrillation, your atria do not contract regularly. So 40% of the effectiveness of your heart muscle as a pump can be lost.

are proven to have a reduced risk of readmission to hospital.[2] On the other hand, recent data show that in certain parts of Canada women are less likely to be referred for specialty heart failure care than men.[3] Being proactive can minimize any potential care gaps for you or your family members.

❤ **You need to know: If you have a diagnosis of heart failure, and your care is being managed solely by your family doctor, you should ask to be referred to a specialist—at least for an evaluation.**

High-Tech Therapies

Cardiac resynchronization therapy (CRT) is a newer intervention used to treat people with heart failure. It has been linked to an improvement of quality of life and may even prolong the lives of patients who have severe heart-muscle damage and are not responding to other therapies. CRT isn't a medication but rather a "device therapy" that essentially uses pacemaker wires to produce a more effective pumping action in the heart. When your heart muscle is weakened, electrical impulses can be delayed, creating inefficiency in the mechanical pumping of the heart. In a CRT procedure, pacemaker leads (wires) are usually inserted into three spots in the heart. Resynchronization means the pacemakers fire to overcome any electrical delays. In other words, they stimulate the electrical activity of the heart.

As stated earlier, if you have an extremely weakened heart muscle, you may also be a candidate for an implantable defibrillator, provided you have been stable for at least six months since your most recent heart failure episode. Implantable defibrillators do not actually treat heart failure. However, they may help people with heart failure survive dangerous

Biventricular Pacemaker for CRT

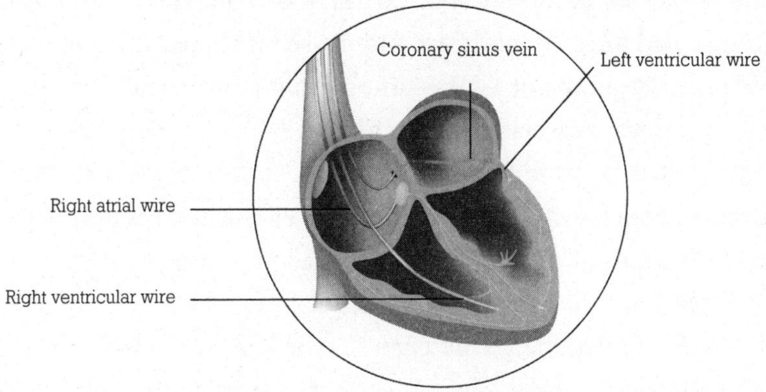

Coronary sinus vein

Left ventricular wire

Right atrial wire

Right ventricular wire

arrhythmias. A defibrillator is a device that is inserted under the skin in your chest. If it detects that the pace of your heartbeats is delayed, disrupted or too fast, the defibrillator will shock the heart into a more steady rhythm (see Chapter 11).

Some patients with heart failure will not require such advanced medical interventions. Rather, they'll be fine managing their disease with medications and lifestyle modifications. That is, if they don't decide to take matters into their own hands. I'm reminded of a lovely 67-year-old patient—a woman who was single, had never married but had a strong support system of friends. This patient was, unfortunately, not in control of her risk factors for cardiovascular disease. She was overweight and had high blood pressure. Most concerning of all, she had stopped her prescription for hypertension medication. Two years before I met her, she simply decided enough was enough. She was sick of taking pills. I suspect she didn't believe they were making any difference. It's a common problem with people who decide to stop their medication: They don't "see" the disease they're preventing, so they mistakenly conclude that there's really nothing wrong with them.

Her family doctor, who suspected she had congestive heart failure, referred her to me. The doctor was right. Her high blood pressure had affected her heart and caused it to weaken. She had common symptoms of CHF—among them an increased shortness of breath, especially when she was lying down, a sense of bloating and extreme fatigue. I worried about my patient. Her ejection fraction—the measure of how well the heart is pumping blood—was at 20%. That's less than half the number it should be. When I saw her, I wanted to admit her to hospital, but she refused. So we negotiated her care. I made it clear she had to take her medications and restrict her sodium. I insisted on seeing her the following week.

Six months later, she was faithfully taking her medications and her heart function had almost returned to normal. She still isn't crazy about taking pills, but with the help of her supporters—a good friend, her family doctor and me—she is managing her condition as best as she can. The important thing is, she is taking her meds. As a person living with high blood pressure and heart failure, she's keeping up her end of the bargain. She's living a longer, healthier life as a result.

13

VALVE SURGERY

"My mom has a narrowed aortic valve, and the doctors say she needs an operation. Is this the same as a bypass surgery?"

The answer is: Not exactly. Certainly, there's a similarity that links a valve operation to a bypass surgery. They're both potentially life-saving procedures. They're also open-heart surgeries, and as such, they are not to be taken lightly. Anyone embarking on a surgery of this magnitude should prepare for weeks to months of recuperation time. If you have ever had major surgery, particularly one in which your chest is pried open, then you know the effects. It's as if a Mack truck has run you over.

It may be terrifying to think of this, but your heart may need to stop pumping in order for your surgeon to operate on it. Don't worry; the surgical team has it under control. To understand why surgeons do this, try to draw a straight line on a constantly moving object. It's nearly impossible. The object has to be kept still. It's the same with your heart. Although some heart operations are done on a beating heart, most of the time your heart is put to sleep. During this time, the blood in your body will be sent to your brain by a mechanical pump.

There are two main types of cardiac valve surgery: aortic and mitral. Both valve surgeries are relatively common. If you or a loved one is scheduled to have valve surgery (or any major surgery), then it is important to know if any other problems need to be addressed. For instance, if you are a patient who is somewhat older and potentially at risk for coronary heart disease, then a coronary angiogram may be performed before any valve surgery. As discussed in Chapter 6, a coronary angiogram is an invasive test to measure blood flow to your heart. Doctors perform the test to see if you have any narrowings or blockages in your arteries. In this case, the surgeon needs to determine if she should perform coronary artery bypass surgery at the same time as your valve surgery, in order to deal with the narrowings in your arteries. She'd rather not go back in a second time for more surgery.

Valve surgery tends to be more complex than coronary artery bypass surgery. Your cardiologist and cardiac surgeon will look at numerous factors: the type of valve problem you have (see Chapter 9), your age, your symptoms and how strong your heart muscle is (based on the ejection fraction). No two patients with valve problems are the same, so you'll have to discuss all the larger and smaller issues related to this surgery with your physician.

❤ **You need to know: Discuss the considerations and implications of valve surgery with your medical team. Be aware of the various issues they're looking at, including what kind of valve problem you have, how well your heart pump is functioning and how your age impacts your surgery.**

Which Type of Valve: Metal or Pig?

Your aortic and mitral valves can be replaced with either a metal, or mechanical, valve or a bioprosthetic valve—that is, a non-metal, artificial valve made from a natural material. Common bioprosthetic valves come from pigs (porcine) or cows (bovine).

If you need a valve replacement, it's important to ask your physician if he is planning to use a metal or pig valve, and what the pros and cons will be in each particular instance. The metal variety tends to last longer, for up to 20 years or more, while pig valves may wear and tear over the years. Patients receiving a metal valve must take blood-thinning medications such as warfarin in order to prevent clots in the valve, as metal is more "sticky" than a natural material. In other words, platelets can adhere to the metal and clots can form.

If you receive a bioprosthetic valve, you do not need to be on blood thinners (warfarin) to protect your valve from clotting. Bioprosthetic valves are often used for patients who are slightly older or have a risk of bleeding. Cardiac surgeons tell me this kind of valve will last for many years longer if used for an older patient compared with a young patient. That is, if you are 40, a non-metal valve may last 10 years before it may wear down, but if you are 65, the same valve may last for 20 years. A younger heart is simply more active and more susceptible to wear and tear.

To decide which type of valve you need, your cardiologist will weigh the length of time the valve will be needed versus the hassle of being on blood-thinning medication. In general, if I have a patient in her 50s who is not at risk for bleeding while taking a blood thinner, I will recommend a metal valve. The patient may need to be on blood thinners anyway—for instance, if she has an irregular heartbeat, specifically a rhythm disturbance called an atrial fibrillation (see Chapter 9). In this case, the metal valve may be the better option.

However, if you are a young woman about to undergo valve surgery and are of child-bearing age, your cardiologist may recommend a pig valve. A bioprosthetic valve will safely get you through your pregnancies, even though it wears out sooner than a metal valve and might have to be replaced again down the road. Talk to your cardiologist about your specific situation.

❤ **You need to know: Although metal valves tend to last longer than natural valves, they require that you take blood thinners regularly to prevent clots from forming.**

If you have had valve surgery of any kind, you should be followed regularly by a cardiologist—usually at least every year or so. Follow-up screening with an echocardiogram (an ultrasound of the heart) is also usually recommended.

Aortic Valve Replacement

You may need your aortic valve replaced most commonly because the valve is too narrow (which is known as aortic stenosis) or, less commonly, because the valve is leaky (known as aortic regurgitation). If you're experiencing shortness of breath, chest pain or fainting and have a very narrowed aortic valve, you may be a candidate for surgery. However, many patients with very narrow aortic valves do not have any symptoms. These individuals need to have their health monitored by the watchful eye of a cardiologist, but they do not require surgery unless their condition changes and symptoms appear.

❤ **You need to know: In general, you need to replace your aortic valve if the vale is very narrow and you are having symptoms of shortness of breath, chest pain or fainting.**

Aortic stenosis tends to occur in both younger patients in their 30s, 40s and even 50s who are born with an abnormal aortic valve and in older patients (usually over age 75) who have developed narrow valves. Younger patients who are born with an abnormal bicuspid aortic valve (see Chapter 1) are at risk of the valve narrowing over time, with wear and tear. Any worn valve may also have calcium buildup.

Cardiologists assess how narrow your valve is by using several measurements. Two of these measurements include (1) the size of the valve area through which the blood flows and (2) the pressure difference across the narrowed area, called a gradient. Severe aortic stenosis is defined as a valve area less than 0.9 cm^2 and/or a gradient of more than 50 mm Hg.

As with any surgery or treatment, you need to weigh the risk of surgery against the benefit. If you have symptomatic aortic stenosis—that is, you have a very narrow valve and are experiencing shortness of breath, fluid on the lungs, chest pain or fainting episodes—the risk of aortic valve replacement is usually outweighed by benefit. This is because your chance of dying from severe aortic stenosis tends to increase drastically the moment you develop symptoms. But before you have symptoms, your risk of having a life-threatening issue because of the valve is not as great as the risk of surgery itself.

Let's now turn to an aortic valve that is leaky (aortic regurgitation). Leaky aortic valves can cause the heart to enlarge (or dilate) over time. If your aortic valve is leaking to the point where your heart is enlarging, you may need to have an aortic valve replacement. You may also need a replacement if there is an enlarging of the aorta, which sits above the valve.

In general, if the aortic valve is damaged to the point of causing harm, the valve should be replaced. We tend to replace—and not to repair—aortic valves since most narrowed aortic valves contain calcium, which makes them difficult for the surgeon to operate on. It's like trying to sew through a piece of hard plastic—a task that is more difficult than sewing through a piece of fabric. Again, these are complex and specialized issues to talk to your cardiologist about.

Mitral Valve Replacement and Repair

A mitral valve replacement is a big heart operation. Compared with other types of heart surgeries, such as aortic valve replacement or coronary artery bypass, mitral valve replacement tends to be slightly more complex. It's also associated with a slightly higher risk of surgery-related complications such as a risk of stroke or even death. If your physician sends you for a mitral valve replacement, the decision has not been made lightly. Mitral valve replacements are performed for either a very narrowed valve (mitral stenosis) or a leaky valve (mitral regurgitation). In either case, usually prior to mitral valve replacement, you'll have experienced symptoms such as difficulty breathing or you may have developed arrhythmias. If these symptoms have not been treated well with medications, you may be a candidate for the surgery. Mitral valve surgery is, despite its complexity, a commonly performed surgery. However, it requires a skilled and experienced surgeon. If you are being considered for mitral valve surgery, ask your cardiologist to recommend a specific surgeon who tends to do more mitral valve surgeries than others.

❤ **You need to know: Mitral valve surgery is a complicated surgery that requires you to be in the hands of an expert surgeon. Ask your cardiologist to refer you to a specific surgeon who has lots of experience with mitral valves.**

It's also possible and, in fact, preferable to perform a repair on the mitral valve—though that's still open-heart surgery. Whether or not you're a candidate for this kind of procedure depends on the complexity of your valve issue and, to some degree, the talents of your surgeon. Your cardiologist will assess your symptoms. He will look at the difficulty you may have in breathing, whether there is increased pressure in your lungs and whether or not you've gone into an irregular heart rhythm (specifically, atrial fibrillation). If your valve is repairable, then your cardiologist may recommend surgery sooner, even in the absence of symptoms. However, if your mitral valve is not easily repaired, then your cardiologist may wait and watch you until you are having severe symptoms before sending you for major valve replacement. As a rule, candidates for mitral valve repair do not usually need to go on long-term blood thinners—unless they're in atrial fibrillation.

❤ **You need to know: The decision to send you for surgery to replace an abnormal mitral valve will depend to some degree on whether or not it will be more easily repaired than replaced.**

Currently, surgeons can't repair a leaky mitral valve without open-heart surgery, unlike repairing a narrowed mitral valve (see the next section), which can be done in a catheterization lab. However, newer technology is evolving that may one day change this (see Chapter 16).

Mitral Valvuloplasty

A valvuloplasty means an opening up of a valve. A narrow mitral valve can sometimes be corrected in a cath lab—a suite in a dedicated cardiac centre where heart procedures, such as angioplasty, are performed. This is not major surgery. Ideal candidates for this procedure will have a narrow valve that is not too thick or encumbered with calcium. During this procedure, a catheter (tube) is inserted into your heart with a deflated balloon at its tip. The catheter is placed through your mitral valve. The balloon is inflated, and your mitral valve is popped open. Although this is performed well in the hands of a skilled cardiologist, mitral valvuloplasty might have adverse consequences, including opening up the valve too much and causing a leaky valve (or mitral regurgitation).

Not all people with mitral stenosis are candidates for mitral valvuloplasty. As cardiologists, we determine the likelihood of success based on the results of an echocardiogram (see Chapter 7). We look to see how much calcium there is in your valve, how thick your valve is and how much your valve moves. If your valve is very thick, has a lot of calcium and doesn't move much, then the likelihood of success in trying to open up your narrowed valve with a balloon procedure is low. In this case, you may need to have open-heart surgery and mitral valve replacement.

In years past, doctors performed a mitral valvuloplasty in an operating room. This was called an open or surgical commissurotomy. Here, the surgeon would open up the mitral narrowing with an instrument or even his fingers. In areas of the developing world, where surgeons do not have the luxury of heart–lung machines and advanced technology, opening up the mitral valve with an open commissurotomy is still effective and useful.

If you have had valve surgery, whether it's an aortic or mitral valve replacement or repair, you should be followed regularly by a cardiologist—at least every year or so. I stress this point because I have seen many patients over the years who are "lost to follow-up." You will benefit from a yearly screening with an echocardiogram to check on the condition of the valve. I had a patient transferred to my care via air ambulance several years ago. She was admitted with congestive heart failure and had a severely weakened heart muscle caused by aortic stenosis. She went on to have life-saving surgery performed by a very skilled surgeon. Six months after the fact, she came to see me for a follow-up. Her heart muscle had returned to normal. Now, she greets me with hugs at her yearly checkup. She and her heart are thriving.

14

SECONDARY PREVENTION AND CARDIAC REHAB

"After her heart attack, my sister's friend was sent to cardiac rehab. I'm not sure what that means. What does rehab involve, and is it really necessary?"

Prevention is a topic I return to time and time again—whether I'm counselling patients one on one, speaking at medical conferences or writing a book. In cardiology, we believe that preventive medicine is absolutely key in treating all heart disease. You have already read about primary prevention (Chapter 4), which are the steps you can take to minimize the likelihood of developing heart disease in the first place. Secondary prevention is just as important and quite similar in its approaches and goals. Secondary prevention involves taking significant steps to ensure you make the right choices *after* you've been diagnosed with heart disease; all the suggestions for primary prevention also apply. Anyone living with heart disease is dealing with a unique set of circumstances, each of which plays a role in your future outlook. Precisely how the disease affects you is influenced by your age, your risk factors and the severity of your condition, in addition to your plan for living with heart disease in a healthy way.

Your circumstances may be different from those of your friends. You may have had an angioplasty for a narrowed coronary artery. You may have had a heart attack, or perhaps you're being treated for stable angina with medications. Each interaction or treatment may bring a different result for each individual. In any event, it's imperative to take your doctor's advice so you can live as long as possible with a good quality of life. Whatever your circumstances, you need to practise secondary prevention—making lifestyle changes and taking medications to keep you from landing in the hospital again. Your goal is to prevent what physicians call a recurrent event: the next heart attack or the next stroke. The risk of a recurrent event is higher if you have coronary heart disease than if you do not. Secondary prevention measures can make a big difference in your quality of life and in your life expectancy.

Cardiac Rehab

Unlike stroke rehab programs, which are designed to help patients regain function, and unlike drug rehab programs, where patients are helped with addictions, cardiac rehab is a comprehensive prevention program designed to allow people to live healthier lives with heart disease.

Cardiac rehab programs vary in style, but they have common and very valuable elements. These include nutrition counselling; smoking cessation; physical activity counselling; exercise training; and counselling for weight management, cholesterol control, management of hypertension (high blood pressure) and dealing with psychosocial issues that may arise after a diagnosis. Ultimately, you'll receive a thorough plan for living a healthy life. Think of it this way: In rehab, doctors provide lifestyle counselling that *everyone* should be taking. If you have had a recent heart attack or have been diagnosed with coronary heart disease, these interventions are all the more important.

In a traditional track-based cardiac rehab program, you will come in to exercise on a track or treadmill several days per week, perhaps at a local community centre. In addition to testing your heart's tolerance for exercise, you will receive education and advice from experts, often nurses.

I run a prevention and rehab program that is not track based. It's located at St. Michael's Hospital in downtown Toronto, where we see patients from all over Ontario. The program is based on a model from Stanford University that uses experts in the field to educate patients, teach them how to exercise and give them an exercise plan to take to their home environment. If you attend my cardiac prevention program, a physician assesses you. You will have a stress test of your heart (see Chapter 6) while you are taking your medications, and you will be given a prescription for exercise based on your stress test results. A dietitian, pharmacist and nurse educator will also see you. All three will give you valuable advice on the daily needs of managing your heart disease. If you smoke, you will receive advice and tools for smoking cessation. Importantly, in this non-traditional rehab program, the physician will assess your heart medications and adjust them as needed.

The benefits of cardiac rehab are similar whether you or your family member attends a traditional track-based rehab program or a non-track-based rehab program. It's simply vital to attend one.

That said, I do want to point out a central issue with cardiac rehab. Despite the proven benefits of rehab, not everyone who should access this level of care does. In fact, studies suggest that less than 20% of all eligible patients with heart disease go on to a cardiac rehab program. In some cases, this may be because your physician believes you are receiving the right medications and lifestyle interventions on your own and don't need rehab. That's dangerous thinking. You can't, in fact, do it all alone—none of us can.

Extensive studies of rehab, each involving more than 10,000 patients followed over the course of six months, prove that patients who attend cardiac rehab have a lower chance of dying from any cause, including from coronary heart disease, than patients who did not go to rehab.[1] Rehab patients also had lower cholesterol levels, lower blood pressure levels and lower rates of smoking than patients who did not attend rehab. So no matter how qualified your cardiologist is, preventive programs are invaluable.

What's more, women are often less likely than men to go to cardiac rehab. There are several reasons why. If you are an older, frailer woman, you may have difficulty securing the transportation to get to your program. Without help, it can be a challenge to make it to doctors' appointments, let alone cardiac rehab. In these cases, arranging for accessible transportation (for example, Wheel-Trans or Handi-Trans) or other organized transportation is essential.

❤ **You need to know:** **Patients are under-referred to cardiac rehab. If you or a family member has had a recent diagnosis of coronary heart disease, ask your doctor for a referral to a rehab program. Patients in cardiac rehab programs have a lower statistical chance of dying from heart disease than patients who have not attended them. No matter how qualified your cardiologist is, she shouldn't treat you in isolation. Rehab is good for your health!**

Treating Depression at Rehab

An important aspect of cardiac rehab and prevention programs is psychosocial support. It's common to experience bouts of depression, fear or anger after a heart attack. Several years ago, a student working with me conducted a psychological survey of patients admitted to the cardiology floor. The results of the survey were shocking. Up to 40% of these heart patients were suffering from some form of depression.

If you have coronary heart disease and you are feeling pessimistic or depressed, you may benefit from supportive therapy and, where necessary, antidepressant medication. Usually, your doctor will help you clarify your fears and frustrations, and your mood will improve within several weeks after a heart attack or a new diagnosis of heart disease. However, sometimes it takes longer to deal with the issues. In fact, in my cardiac prevention and rehab program, we screen patients for depression throughout their care because it is so common.

❤ **You need to know: Depression is common after a heart attack. If your mood is down or you feel angry after a heart attack, these are often signs of depression. It's important that you talk to your doctor about this. If necessary, you may be prescribed medications for depression that are effective and safe for heart patients.**

Our rehab team at St. Michael's Hospital includes a cardiac psychiatrist trained to help people deal with depression in the face of medical illness. Many patients benefit from this resource. You can also cope with depression by discussing your fears with friends, family members and other health care professionals. If you or a family member notices that you have become angrier or more frustrated after a diagnosis of a heart attack, that's often a sign of depression. It's important that you talk to your doctor about any such feelings you may be experiencing. If you have been diagnosed with depression and are living with coronary heart disease, you can access safe, effective mood-lifting medications that will not interfere with your heart pills or your future risk of heart disease. Remember that your mental health is as important as your physical health!

Returning to Work

Whether or not you're physically ready to return to work after a heart attack depends on the amount of heart-muscle damage you experienced and the type of work you perform.

In many cases, you can return to work faster than you think. Years ago, when we did not have the kind of advanced and successful treatments that are now commonplace in cardiology, you were more likely to be left with extensive heart-muscle damage after a heart attack. You may have stayed in a hospital for several weeks. Fortunately, we're a lot more efficient these days. In fact, you may come to the emergency room with chest pain, have a mild abnormality show up in your blood tests or ECG and go right on to further testing such as an angiogram and then a procedure such as an angioplasty. Nowadays, most patients are discharged from hospital within a few days of their angioplasty or even their heart attack. If this is the case, and there has been very little heart-muscle damage, your ability to return to work is usually not an issue.

After a Small Heart Attack

If you have a desk job, it's not dangerous from a physical perspective to return to work after a small heart attack. Precisely when to return—whether it's a week or two after you leave the hospital, or even longer—is a matter to discuss with your physician. Everyone has different capacities and circumstances.

However, if you had a moderate amount of heart-muscle damage and you are a construction worker whose job entails lifting heavy objects, returning to work could prove risky. If you have a physically demanding job, consult your doctor to evaluate the impact that work will have on your health. Sudden exertion can be dangerous, so it's possible you may no longer be able to work in the same job or at the same intensity as before.

I find that patients or their family members are often fearful of returning to work. Many times, however, they will do better psychologically once they get back to their normal routines. But it's also not healthy to return to a job the day after an angioplasty without acknowledging that you have had a serious, potentially life-threatening problem. Patients need time to pause and reflect. Balance is key.

After a Large Heart Attack or Major Surgery

If you worked before you had a significant heart attack or surgery, you can usually go back to the same job within 8 to 16 weeks, according to the Heart and Stroke Foundation's Road to Recovery guidelines. How soon you can return depends on many factors including your symptoms, how you feel and the physical demands or stresses of your job. It may be a good idea to return to work on a part-time basis at first and gradually work up to full-time hours. If you are close to retirement age, you may not want to return to work at all. You may rather spend more time with your friends and family pursuing hobbies or interests you enjoy, or engage in volunteer work. You may be eligible for a retirement pension, employment insurance or a disability pension. To help find out what benefits you are eligible for, you can talk with a social worker, a human resources manager or your boss.

One aspect of returning to work involves looking at the lifestyle you led before your heart attack. Were you working 16-hour days in your job? Did your exercise routine fall by the wayside? Did you turn to fast foods because you didn't have any time to cook? It's not the stress in your life that will kill you but how you deal with stress. The habits you form in stressful periods have an impact, whether you're reaching for that greasy burger or giving up your morning walk in order to squeeze in just another hour on the laptop. I recommend that you take some time to reflect on how you were living your life before your heart attack. Were you simply stuck in the rat race, or did you take time for yourself to lead a healthy and happy life?

After a heart attack, not everyone needs to have a profound revelation, quit a stressful job and join a yoga colony in India. However, most of us will need to establish a sense of balance after we are diagnosed with a serious, and potentially life-threatening, disease. In some cases, you may feel you've been given a chance to open a new career chapter. Although switching jobs can be exciting, it can also bring new stresses. Talk to your friends and family to help and support you in making a change if necessary.

❤ **You need to know: You should discuss your readiness to return to work with your physician. It is usually physically safe to return to work even several days after a small heart attack, but you should take at least a week or so off work to pause and reflect on what has happened. If you have had a significant heart attack, however, you may not be able to return to work right away and in some cases not at all.**

Over the years, many patients have told me they feel too fatigued after a heart attack and are unable to go back to work. Extreme fatigue after a heart attack usually occurs only if you have significant heart-muscle damage. Sometimes, medications such as beta blockers can cause fatigue—although with newer drugs, this is much less common than it used to be. However, the most common cause of fatigue after a heart attack is psychological. I'm not suggesting it's "all in your head," but unless you have significant heart-muscle damage, fatigue is *not* a common consequence of a recent heart attack. Anxiety and stress are common causes of fatigue. Talk to your doctor and family about your fears and concerns.

❤ **You need to know: The most common cause of fatigue after a heart attack is psychological—something you and your physician can deal with!**

Beyond Work: Resuming Your Routine After a Major Heart Attack or Surgery

When should you get back to your regular activities at home? I'm asked that question all the time. According to the Heart and Stroke Foundation's *Road to Recovery* guidelines, it's important to proceed in stages after you return home following a large heart attack or open-heart surgery.

In weeks one through three at home, you can start by taking a few steps outside and doing light housework. That said, I encourage anyone dealing with a new diagnosis to pass the work baton immediately. Enlist help for household activities. Engage in hobbies or activities you can do when sitting down, such as reading or crafts. Climb one flight of stairs slowly, and walk around your house or yard as instructed by your cardiac rehab team or doctor. You can ride as a passenger in a car for short trips of about half an hour. You can make social visits. Also, you can lift up to 5 pounds (2.5 kg) of any kind of weight.

Three to six weeks after your heart attack or hospitalization, you can continue walking as instructed by your physician or rehab team. You may also resume sexual relations once you are able to climb two flights of stairs, but avoid sex if you have had a large meal or alcohol or are feeling tired—these can divert blood flow from your heart. You can also make more social visits, work a little in the garden, shop for groceries or perform light housework. But again I would encourage you to get others to do chores you do not want to do. At this point, you can lift up to 10 pounds (5 kg), ride in a car for up to one hour and, if approved by your doctor, drive, dance slowly, fish, sail a small boat, cycle at medium speed, play table tennis or go five-pin bowling.

After six weeks, you can resume all normal levels of activity such as walking at a brisk pace, cycling, cross-country skiing, skating, swimming, and lifting or carrying up to 20 pounds (10 kg); you can return to work with your doctor's approval. You can also golf, starting with nine holes, providing you play during the cooler parts of the day in the summer months and use a golf cart to carry your clubs. With all activity, go at your own pace, and rest when necessary.[2]

Whatever your circumstances, the Heart and Stroke Foundation reminds people that you need to take some time for yourself. Ask family members, friends and neighbours to help you with errands, child care, shopping, yardwork, cooking and cleaning the house. Remember, getting others to help you when you need it most is not likely to be permanent. You are not "a failure" if you rely on others. This mentality may take a little getting used to if you are a type A personality and are used to doing everything yourself.

It's important for you to individualize your recovery; resume activity when the time is right. Each of us is different and has varied interests and abilities. In fact, I have never *actually* advised my patients to do a specific activity—whether it's to take up five-pin bowling, table tennis or golf. Most often, I encourage them to get outside of the house with a friend and simply start moving again. If you are diagnosed with heart disease, my advice is just to *start* a regular activity routine. Many patients are not that active prior to surgery or a massive heart attack. After they recover, they need to become active—get off the couch and do something!

Never Again

There are some things my patients living with heart disease can never do again. Shovelling snow is one of them. This task is actually quite dangerous because it involves abrupt exertion: It's not a type of physical activity that allows you to build up your heart rate gradually. In addition, you're pushing or lifting heavy loads when you shovel snow, and you're doing it in cold weather. Cold air constricts the blood vessels, which has the exact opposite effect of nitroglycerine (a spray or tablet medication taken for coronary artery disease that opens up, or dilates, the blood vessels). If you are living in a cold climate, you may need to pay someone younger who lives around the corner to help you clear the snow. This is one of my rules to which I have no exception!

On the other hand, you may be able to gradually build up to doing other physical activity such as repetitive work with your arms in warmer weather (raking the leaves, cutting the grass or vacuuming). Clearly, how you increase your physical activity needs to be discussed with your doctor or your cardiac rehab team.

Driving

When is it safe to return to driving after a heart attack? The short answer is that it's complicated. In some provinces and in parts of the United States, it's illegal for you to drive for a month after a heart attack. If your licence is revoked after a heart attack, it can become a bureaucratic nightmare for physicians and patients alike. Getting your licence reinstated is often a lengthy battle involving stacks of paperwork.

On the other hand, some patients should simply not be driving because they are at risk of having a recurrent heart attack or of developing a sudden arrhythmia (when the heart beats too fast) and collapse. You would not want to be behind a wheel and lose consciousness, putting yourself and others at risk.

The Canadian Cardiovascular Society advises[3] that whether you can drive after a heart attack is based on your future risk for additional problems and the type of driving you do. For this reason, the advice is a general rule of thumb. The recommendation is that if you've had a large heart attack, where a blood clot completely occluded (or blocked off) the coronary artery and you had significant heart-muscle damage, you can resume private driving one month after discharge, provided you have received clot-busting medications or angioplasty. You can start commercial driving three months after discharge for this type of heart attack. After bypass surgery, the general recommendation is to wait for one month to drive after you have been discharged and sent home.

If you've had a small heart attack that has not left you with significant heart-muscle damage, you may drive two days after having an angioplasty procedure. If you did not receive angioplasty, you can drive seven days after discharge.

If you have stable coronary disease and stable angina (see Chapter 8), or if you do not have symptoms but have been diagnosed with coronary disease in general, there are no restrictions on driving. If you have chronic coronary artery disease, you should wait two days after an angioplasty is performed before driving.

Driving after you've been diagnosed with a serious rhythm problem, however, is another story. In general, if you have previously collapsed from a life-threatening arrhythmia (such as ventricular tachycardia; see Chapter 9), your licence should be revoked. You can't start thinking about driving for personal reasons until six months after the event. If you are a commercial driver—for example, a truck driver or school bus driver—you may be disqualified from this work forever.

If you or a family member has received a pacemaker, we generally wait a week to allow you to drive. Patients with internal implantable defibrillators (see Chapter 11) usually are restricted from driving for between one and six months and even longer, depending on whether the defibrillator is being activated. (A defibrillator becomes active when it senses the heart is in a dangerous rhythm disturbance.)

❤ **You need to know: Driving after a serious arrhythmia is a different matter than driving after a heart attack or heart procedure. If you have collapsed from a life-threatening rhythm problem, in general, your licence should be revoked.**

One of the problems that physicians and patients face is that medical recommendations are not always reflected in the law, and laws vary in different jurisdictions. Sometimes physicians will revoke licences for legitimate medical and legal reasons. Unfortunately, reinstating the licence after the appropriate time has passed can be difficult. This is an issue I believe the public, physicians and governments will need to address at some point. I see patients who are very frustrated because it is actually a longer process to reinstate a licence than to take it away.

When to See Your Doctor

In an ideal world, you would have easy access to your cardiologist and specialists at all hours of the day and night so you could ask questions and alleviate your fears. Realistically, that's not possible in any modern health care system. That doesn't mean you can't be proactive about your health. I encourage you to play an active advocacy role in your health care and make sure you are dealing with a physician who provides thorough answers to your questions. Even in my busy practice, my assistant passes on all messages, and I return all calls within a reasonable amount of time.

Talk to your doctor if you are thinking about stopping your prescription medication. This may sound obvious, but even the most educated patients need to be reminded how dangerous it is to cease taking their pills. I had put one of my patients, a lawyer, on a plan to take various rhythm medications for his arrhythmia. This plan included staying on medications for two months, seeing me in my office and then deciding whether he needed an electrical cardioversion (a procedure that changes the rhythm of your heart from abnormal to normal; see Chapter 11). I had organized his follow-up appointment so that the timing would allow for his medication to take effect. Unfortunately, two weeks after seeing me initially, he decided he noticed no difference in how he felt on or off the medications. He then stopped the medications without telling his doctors. At the two-month follow-up appointment, I had to start from scratch with his medication plan. Had he left a message with my office to let me know what was going on, I would have seen him sooner and advised him to continue the medication.

It's important after an initial diagnosis of heart disease that you and your family members write down a list of questions to discuss with your cardiologist—particularly after your hospital discharge. Writing down your questions will both focus the issue and make sure the valuable time you do have with your doctor is well spent. Sometimes health care professionals such as a dietitian or pharmacist in your cardiac rehab program can better address certain questions regarding lifestyle changes. Nonetheless, you should always ask.

It is especially important to talk to your doctor if you experience a change in mood after a diagnosis of heart disease or a recent heart attack, or if you are experiencing discomfort that recurs after discharge from hospital. It's not uncommon for you to experience aches and pains that you did not have before your heart attack. Often, once you have been through a serious situation and admitted to hospital for a heart attack, your brain will play tricks on your body. This is different from experiencing an actual recurrence of heart attack symptoms such as chest, arm, throat or jaw discomfort, which occurs when your heart cries out for blood in the same way it did during the first attack. You should seek medical attention if you feel a return of heart attack symptoms or discomfort, even if it's on a smaller scale.

❤ **You need to know: Unless you are examined by your doctor, it may be difficult for you to sort out if your pain is coming from your heart or not. In general, sharp, stabbing, pinpoint pains that last several seconds are usually not worrisome and not related to the heart.**

If you or a family member is having new, severe chest pains that feel similar to your heart attack, go straight to the emergency room. If, on the other hand, the discomfort occurs with exertion and goes away with rest, then it is reasonable to leave a phone message with your physician and wait for his advice on the next steps. Even if we all seem connected by iPhones and BlackBerrys, sending an email to your doctor to say you're having chest pain is *not* the right approach.

I'm reminded of a tragic story that occurred when I first went into practice. I had a patient with severe coronary heart disease. He was on the right medications and doing reasonably well until, one day, he developed severe chest pain. Instead of calling 9-1-1 and seeking urgent medical attention, his daughter emailed me. Unfortunately, doctors have multiple demands on their schedules and cannot be on email all the time. They can be on call, seeing patients and away from their computers or even unable to scroll through their BlackBerrys. The email arrived at 10:00 a.m., but I did not check my email until 1:00 that afternoon. I called right back and told them to call 9-1-1. Unfortunately the patient had experienced a massive heart attack and had lost three valuable hours since the initial chest pain. My patient did not survive. If you have an urgent problem, then calling an ambulance is the best thing to do.

❤ **You need to know: In business, the saying is "Time is money." In cardiology, we say, "Time is heart muscle." If you are potentially having a heart attack, seek urgent medical attention or your heart muscle may be irreparably damaged. Don't send out an email asking your cardiologist what to do. Get to the emergency room!**

You should consult your doctor if you have symptoms after you've been discharged from the hospital. The following are warning signs:

- You experience angina (chest discomfort) with low activity or when resting.
- You wake up at night with angina.
- You have more frequent or severe bouts of angina.
- You have to take nitroglycerine more often than usual to relieve symptoms of chest discomfort, or you need to take more nitroglycerine because it does not work as quickly as it used to.
- You experience shortness of breath.
- You notice your ankles or legs are swollen.
- You feel light-headed, you've fainted or you experience a racing or pounding heart.

Likelihood of Recurrence

As soon as you have a heart attack, your future risk of a recurrent heart attack is greater than someone who doesn't have heart disease. Your greatest risk for a life-threatening problem exists in the initial few days after the heart attack; then your risk decreases after a month, and it drops again over time. You can lessen the likelihood of a recurrence by controlling your risk factors and being on appropriate medication. The risk is greatest, however, if you continue to smoke or have uncontrolled diabetes. High blood pressure or high cholesterol will also put you at a greater risk for recurrent heart attacks. Age plays a part too. Your risk of dying after a heart attack can be as high as 20% if you are over age 80 (compared with less than 5% in men 50 and under).

There's no doubt that heart disease can be deadly, but fortunately, the kind of cardiac care now available to patients is far more advanced than it used to be. In fact, when I was a resident 20 years ago, the first studies evaluating blood thinners for unstable angina were nicknamed "the Montreal Death Trials." (The lead cardiologist on the study lived in Montreal.) At that time, the risk of dying in the first six months after a heart attack was as high as 30%. Times have changed, and death rates after a heart attack are now much lower.

A year after a heart attack, if you have not had major heart-muscle damage and are stable and taking current recommended medications, your risk of a major adverse cardiac event is generally less than 2%.[4]

Yes, heart disease can be deadly, but if you or your family member has survived a heart attack, is receiving good care and is on the right medications, then the odds are in your favour that you or your family member will not have a recurrent heart attack or future cardiac issues. For every 100 patients who receive expert and timely care following their diagnosis and are sent on to cardiac rehab programs, 98 will not have a future problem with the disease. However, you are in jeopardy if you have high blood pressure, diabetes or high cholesterol and you are not taking steps to control these conditions. You are certainly at risk if you continue to smoke, which is perilous in so many ways. If you have kidney disease, you also have a higher likelihood of experiencing a future heart attack or stroke than cardiac patients who do not have kidney disease.

I believe it's important, ultimately, to dwell on the positive. In North America, and in Canada especially, we have access to terrific cardiologists and specialized cardiac rehab programs. If you are faced with a diagnosis of heart disease, take advantage of the vast support network that you and your loved ones can access.

15

RELATIONSHIPS AND LIVING WITH HEART DISEASE

"I made a good recovery from my heart attack. But weeks have passed, I still don't feel like myself, and I'm always short tempered with my family. What can I do about this?"

Modern medicine is evolving and advancing all the time. The more innovative medicine becomes, however, the higher the expectations patients have for the level of care they receive. There's a common belief that doctors and hospitals can "fix" almost anything, including your heart. Many patients see the heart as a matter of mechanics—a collection of cells, muscles, valves and arteries that can always be repaired if they are damaged. When that doesn't happen as quickly or as fully as we expect, our capacity to feel emotionally overwhelmed by the disease may increase. Of course, recuperating from a heart attack or living with heart disease is not a matter of quick fixes. Although cardiac care is remarkably sophisticated—and physicians offer a high level of expertise in order to steer the ship of patient care—recovering from a heart attack or major surgery takes time.

That's especially true when it comes to untangling and processing the disease's emotional stresses. Your closest relationships can become greatly affected by a family member's diagnosis of heart disease. Many times this is for the better: A diagnosis can become the epiphany moment that inspires you and your loved ones to live a healthier, more active life. However, even in the best scenarios, physical stresses come hand in hand with psychological ones. After you have a heart attack, for instance, your partner may be afraid of causing harm to you during sex, or you may feel a sense of depression in response to your diagnosis. Let's talk about the areas that may be affected by your anxieties and fears—and what you and your family can do about them.

Relationships and Sex

When it comes to intimacy following a heart attack, surgery or new cardiac diagnosis, it's important to start slowly and communicate your fears and anxieties to your partner and your doctor.

Your physical readiness for sex after a heart attack depends on how severely your heart muscle was damaged and how physically fit you are. Every case is different, but by and large, most people who have not had significant muscle damage after a heart attack can go back to healthy, normal sex lives relatively quickly.

You may feel uncertain about resuming sexual activity and may even think that sex can harm you. Let me assure you that it's very rare for sexual intercourse to bring on a heart attack. Sex is not as demanding on your heart as you may think. In fact, if you can easily walk up two flights of stairs or walk briskly, your heart can usually meet the demands of sexual activity.

You and your partner can discuss personal issues like this one with a support team of medical professionals in a cardiac prevention and rehab program. There, your readiness for physical activity, including sex, will be assessed. Generally, patients attending rehab should be able to perform the second stage of exercise in a test called the Bruce protocol. This diagnostic test is used to evaluate your cardiac function. If you can exercise to the second part of the test (stage 2)—that is, you can walk for more than three minutes on a treadmill without chest pain—then sex is safe. Your electrocardiogram reading must also be in the normal range during the exercise. When your heart can handle this exercise stress, you're usually okay to have sex.

Keep in mind that it's always a good idea to start slowly. For example, it would be unreasonable to proceed with sexual relations with your partner the day you are discharged after your heart attack. In fact, I'd consider you to be in denial about your condition. Build up to an appropriate level of intimacy and physical activity over time. It's valuable to acknowledge that intimacy takes on all forms—including hand-holding, walking and talking and does not necessarily equal the initiation of sexual activity.

♥ **You need to know: If you have had a small heart attack and can walk on a treadmill for three to six minutes, you should be fine physically to return to sexual activity.**

Most people can usually resume sexual activity within two or three weeks of coming home from the hospital. Some heart medications may reduce your sex drive (see Chapter 10), so it may be the case that some men find it more difficult to obtain or maintain an erection. Talk to your doctor if this happens to you.

According to the Heart and Stroke Foundation's *Road to Recovery* guide (www.heartandstroke.ca), it's better to plan in advance for intimacy. Choose times when you and your partner are rested and relaxed, and set aside plenty of time to allow for slowed sexual responses. If you are a woman experiencing vaginal dryness because of heart medications or hormonal changes, try using a water-soluble lubricant such as K-Y jelly. It's a good idea to avoid alternative herbal medications to restore your sexual function or interest. Many herbs interact with medications commonly prescribed for heart disease (see Chapter 10).

Medication for Erectile Dysfunctions

One of the issues with drugs that enhance male sexual performance is that they function by opening up the blood vessels. These drugs are vasodilators. When a man's blood vessels are open, he's able to maintain an erection. However, vasodilators also relax blood vessels elsewhere in the body. When your vessels are relaxed, your blood pressure can fall. One of the big concerns with Viagra-like medications is their interaction with nitroglycerine. You can have an adverse reaction if you take sexual performance–enhancing medication with nitroglycerine, a drug that dilates the blood vessels to relieve chest pain. If you take both drugs, you're magnifying the vasodilation effect and can have a significant drop in blood pressure, so much so that it can potentially be fatal. Although many of my patients wish to take Viagra, I usually do not prescribe the medication to them if they have intermittent angina (chest pain) requiring nitroglycerine, have very low blood pressure or are not able to demonstrate moderate exercise capacity on the treadmill. However, if you are clinically stable, do not have angina requiring nitroglycerine and have good exercise tolerance on the treadmill, Viagra-like drugs are not likely to endanger your health.

Beyond Sex

Relationship issues go well beyond sexual intimacy. If you are living with heart disease, you may confront some frustrating reactions to your condition. By nature, your loved ones are going to worry about you. It's great to have the care and attention, but at

As a rule, don't overdo it. Start slowly. It's the best way to approach sexual intimacy and physical activity. This especially applies if you are older or your fitness level is low. Years ago, at the start of my medical career, I was on call in a hospital when an 83-year-old man came in with a heart attack. I'll never forget what happened next. We were in the midst of giving him clot-busting medications when his very distraught wife pulled me aside. She was hysterical. I found out why: She thought she had almost killed him. His heart attack began while they were attempting to be sexually intimate for the first time in many years. He had also taken Viagra. I reassured his wife that it was not her fault, and that this might have happened anyway, but this was only partially true. They shouldn't have used medications to help them sexually, especially since he was on blood pressure pills and nitroglycerine. He also hadn't seen his doctor in a while. In general, patients who are older, more frail or out of shape should work their way up to having vigorous sexual activity.

times, it can also become stifling. One of my long-time patients was a woman in her 60s who had never married and lived with her well-meaning sister, who was also single. They weren't just siblings but close friends and companions. One day, my patient pulled me aside and told me her sister was driving her crazy because she wouldn't let her take the stairs or perform even minor chores. During one appointment, I had to sit down and play counsellor with the sisters—explaining that it was okay for my patient to resume her activities, even if that meant housework.

It's common for family members to become more protective of you than they need to be. They often fear that your health is so delicate you will easily hurt yourself. More often than not, however, being overprotective has the opposite desired effect—it can actually get in the way of a healthy recovery. I have several patients, for instance, whose family members are fearful of them walking up and down stairs. If it were up to their families, my patients would be entirely sedentary. For recovery to succeed, it's important for everyone to understand that you can go back to a reasonably normal routine. This includes engaging in appropriate physical activity.

Over the years, I've learned that family members can be more devastated by a cardiac event than the patients themselves. I make a point during a cardiac rehab visit to "prove" how well patients are doing by inviting their family members to watch them exercise on the treadmill. They may be reassured to see their spouse, parent or sibling exercise without experiencing chest pain, shortness of breath or an abnormal ECG result.

Being a Caregiver *and* a Patient

We all deal with many conflicting demands on our time, either at home or at work. Most of us are familiar with multi-tasking, and some of us think we're pretty good at the daily juggle (this may be true only in our minds). As the saying goes, if you want to get something done, give it to someone busy. The joke around my house is that I can handle three things at once, but give me four and I'm pushed over the edge.

I've learned over the years, however, that taking on too much will only drain me. So will being a caregiver to everyone around you when you really need to focus on being a patient. Not long ago, I was caring for a woman who needed bypass surgery. To my great dismay, she wanted to put the surgery off. She explained that her husband needed to be in surgery at the same time. However, his procedure was an elective operation. She had a life-threatening heart condition. Despite my protests, she wanted to postpone her bypass. I'm not sure if it was denial that drove her decision making or the fact that she was a classic type E—everything to everyone except herself. Either way, she wasn't prioritizing herself. I did finally convince her to have the surgery. She resolved to go through with it only after she made two weeks of dinners and froze them for her husband. As it turns out, he had never prepared a meal on his own. I'm sure he would have gotten along fine, but her type E personality prevailed.

I have another patient who is a high-achieving 56-year-old professional. As a high-flyer at work, she rarely has enough downtime. She had been battling a weight problem, and her high blood pressure needed to be controlled by medication. For a time, she made a commitment to making a positive change—she joined a healthy eating program, hired a personal trainer and took yoga classes. Then at a certain point, as she became preoccupied with two upcoming projects, all the good effort fell by the wayside. She was, in the end, definitive: "It's not in my vocabulary to take time for myself," she told me. We've all been there from time to time, but behind the words is a deeply concerning mindset. Ultimately, I was forced to increase this patient's medications to reduce her risk of heart attack and stroke, a course of events that could have been prevented if she'd only rewritten her vocabulary—and the rules that govern her life.

My advice is simple to anyone who is living with a new diagnosis of coronary heart disease: Form heart-healthy habits. Take time for yourself. Let people take care of you. Shed some obligations. Delegate work to others. Re-evaluate your tendency to say yes to every demand. Ask a friend or a family member to help you with tasks such as cooking or shopping or yardwork. Slow down, take time for yourself and take time off work, even if it is not medically necessary for you to be away from the office. You may be physically able to go back to work but still tender emotionally. Make sure you've recovered from a psychological point of view before you go back to potentially stress-filled situations.

If you've survived a heart attack, you may be inspired to re-evaluate the choices you've made in the past so you can prioritize your health in the future. Not everyone needs a "big picture" rethink of their lives, but in the short term, a little reflection is essential. Think about how you want to be remembered by your close friends and family. No one wants their tombstone to read: "Never missed a day of work, was a loyal company employee, published 400 papers."

Your Family Members' Fears

If you are living with heart disease, you may have anxieties and concerns that will hopefully be addressed by your health care providers. However, your family members may have their own fears and concerns about your heart disease—issues that are often neglected. You should ask your spouse, children or siblings to discuss what's on their minds at a meeting with your doctor. Communication and knowledge will often solve many problems that might burden your loved ones or even get in the way of your recovery.

Often, family members feel they are losing control after a loved one has had a heart attack. There are some things we cannot control. Sometimes the concerns are related to other personal circumstances, such as a fear of losing not only a loved one but also the primary income earner of the family, which may threaten the family's financial security. I'm a strong believer in sharing your thoughts with a professional as well as your family members. Talk your way through any emotions you may be experiencing. At the same time, encourage your family to focus on the things that are in their control—such as the steps they can take to become healthier and more active, as you are doing the same.

Even though some patients have a genetic predisposition for developing heart disease, much of the disease is related to lifestyle. Our spouses and partners often share the healthy or unhealthy lifestyles we lead. Relatives who visit heart patients in hospital are likely to have multiple risk factors for heart disease themselves.

The good news is that family and friends make for an invaluable and often motivated support team. It can be inspiring to see your family members making the effort alongside you to reduce their risk for heart disease. If they share your heart-healthy lifestyle choices, then it becomes easier for you to make a lasting, positive impact on your own health. Your home is a healthier environment when there is a team approach to healthy eating and healthy living—whether you have heart disease or not.

PART V

Looking to the Future

16

INNOVATIONS

"My son read on the Internet that my mother doesn't really need major bypass surgery for her heart. They can manage her condition with modern medications alone. Is this true?"

Only a generation ago, it was unthinkable that this could be true. However, recent studies suggest that medications alone can treat certain serious heart conditions that used to require surgery. Such is the nature of modern medicine.

It's estimated that every five years, the volume of medical knowledge doubles. So by my calculations, since I graduated from medical school, my knowledge as a physician has multiplied 16 times. That's not to say that everything I learned many years ago is now obsolete. Rather, a wealth of added technologies; new techniques, practices, studies and medications; and general wisdom has emerged to help us prevent, treat and ultimately cure disease and disability.

What does the future hold? Let's look at the latest concepts for the prevention and treatment of heart disease—as well as the obstacles to overcome on the road to scientific progress.

How Newer Drugs Are Tested

More important than knowing about the newest fad treatment in cardiology is the ability to recognize what makes a new medical recommendation credible. As a rule, understanding how cardiologists conduct research will help you better digest information on how to take care of your heart in the future.

Allow me to sketch it out for you. We can have different levels of "evidence" in medicine. Researchers routinely propose a hypothesis about the efficacy of a drug or a surgery. Sometimes their ideas may seem credible, but when the research is evaluated in a proper study, the promises begin to fade. Classic examples include the early observational studies suggesting (erroneously, as it turns out) that hormone replacement therapy can protect women against heart disease. These studies involved watching many thousands of women on HRT. Initially, the observations seemed to suggest that hormones protected the women from developing heart disease. However, in a later properly designed study to evaluate the effects of HRT, this benefit was no longer seen. The reasons these women didn't develop heart disease had nothing to do with the HRT treatment—it was more likely that the women who chose to take HRT were also leading healthier lives.

Most of the advice I've given in this book is based on the principles of evidence-based medicine. This means there are hard factual data to support the use of a particular drug or treatment plan. The only way researchers can determine if a treatment will be effective for the majority of patients is to study the treatment in a randomized controlled trial (or RCT). In an RCT, patients are randomly assigned a drug that is being studied. Usually half of the patients in the study will receive the medication, and the other half will receive a placebo, or fake pill. In a double-blind randomized placebo controlled trial, both the patient and the person handing out the medication are "blind" to the intervention. They do not know who is receiving the real drug and who is receiving the placebo. You may think this sounds unethical but it's not. In fact, if a physician or nurse knows who is receiving what, he may unintentionally be biased in interpreting a patient's symptoms. Well-designed trials are conducted under the supervision of governing bodies, known as data and safety monitoring committees.

What has the research uncovered in cardiology? Recent randomized trials have shown that certain drugs that raise HDL (good cholesterol) are ineffective at lowering your future risk of heart attack. On the other hand, clinical trials have shown that statin drugs that lower LDL (bad cholesterol) are effective at lowering your future risk. So is transcatheter aortic valve implantation (TAVI), a new procedure to replace an aortic valve (see the next section).

Women tend to be under-represented in clinical trials, often because they tend not to volunteer to be studied. Over the years in my practice, I have encouraged my patients who are women, and especially older women who may be excluded in scientific data, to participate in randomized controlled trials. If you or a family member has been approached to potentially participate in a clinical trial, think about it. Obviously no one will twist your arm, but in this day and age, the only studies that are conducted have passed a very high bar for safety and ethical considerations.

The Latest Valve Techniques

In the last few years, there's been an explosion of technological advances for patients with heart valve problems. A narrowed aortic valve, or aortic stenosis, is very common in elderly individuals. I have seen many patients in their 80s go through open-heart valve surgery, but now doctors are evaluating a new, less-invasive technique. It's called transcatheter aortic valve implantation. Known by the acronym TAVI, it's performed in specialized centres under the guidance of both an interventional cardiologist and a surgeon. During a TAVI procedure, you are given a general anesthetic and a surgeon inserts catheters towards your heart, often through the blood vessels. The technique is similar to a coronary angiogram. In a TAVI, the aortic valve is essentially "crushed" open, and then a stent valve—a valve on a wire strut—is inserted in its place.

In the next decade, as TAVI becomes more common, we'll see more information on its long-term outcomes and benefits. In the meantime, my personal prediction is that TAVI is here to stay. Recent data suggest that if you are not a candidate for traditional surgery, TAVI will improve your quality of life and decrease the likelihood that you will be hospitalized for heart disease in the future.[1] However, TAVI is not for everyone. Unfortunately, if you are extremely elderly and frail, you may not be a candidate for TAVI. Physically small patients are also not candidates, since the special valves used in this procedure suit patients of average height or taller. If you or a loved one has aortic stenosis and is older (over 80) or has other health issues that would preclude traditional aortic valve replacement, talk to your cardiologist about TAVI. It can't hurt to be assessed.

♥ You need to know: If you are not a good candidate for aortic valve surgery, ask your doctor for a referral to a centre that performs TAVI, a procedure that is on the cutting edge of cardiac care. Find out if the procedure is right for you.

Gene Therapy: Regenerating the Heart and Blood Vessels

In recent years, the scientific community has made a concerted effort to study ways to regenerate heart muscle after it has been damaged and to regenerate coronary arteries (angiogenesis) after they have become diseased. This is called gene therapy for the heart. Trials are ongoing, and to date this area remains experimental. The general concept behind gene therapy is that your genes, which control cell growth, can be manipulated outside of the body. The genes may be put inside a cell, often in a test tube, and then put back into your body. By and large, researchers will use viruses to enable this process, but these viruses need to be safe. The problem is that it's complicated to transfer the genes into the body. As well, these genes need to target very specific cells. As it stands, researchers need to overcome significant safety hurdles before this becomes a common practice. In fact, many research programs looking at gene therapy have been stopped because of safety concerns for patients. Currently there is no safe and proven way to regenerate blood vessels and heart-muscle cells for everyday cardiac care. In our lifetimes, we may see this new therapy work, but for now, we have other methods, such as medication and preventive steps, to protect ourselves and our families from heart attack and stroke.[2]

Genomics

Your genetic makeup has a significant influence on your health, so knowing your exact DNA may help predict if you are at risk for heart disease or its contributors, diabetes and high blood pressure. This concept sounded like science fiction when I was in medical school, but the area is innovating quickly. In 2001, the Human Genome Project completed a rough draft of all the genes in the human body.[3] By 2007, scientists had mapped the details for the genes—the sequences that make us human beings. These data will now allow researchers to consider the associations between the sequences and diseases. I do believe that in my lifetime, scientists will have the ability to "screen your genes" for disease. In the future, the information our genes provide will be used to treat, and not just screen for, heart disease. Genomics will allow doctors to decide the best type of medication for each of their patients.

In fact, we are already looking at how your genes will predict the effectiveness of certain Aspirin-like drugs for patients after a heart attack. Genomics are also allowing us to discover treatments at a faster pace than ever. We're not quite there yet, but stay tuned—science fiction may become reality before we know it.

The Future Is You: Commit to a Heart-Healthy Life

Ultimately, the best way to look forward is with optimism. With advanced medicine, skilled medical professionals and informed patients, the future is encouraging for many of you living with cardiovascular disease.

The best partner a cardiologist can have is a committed patient. Your success depends on the essential relationship between you and your doctor, which requires the elements of mutual honesty, frequent dialogue and, ultimately, trust in the medical process. You have to believe there's a proven path to follow that will lead you either to be healthier or to manage heart disease in the most effective way possible. In each visit you have with a doctor, whether it's a routine checkup, an appointment in cardiac rehab or a visit to the hospital, keep the line of inquiry alive. Ask plenty of specific questions. You now have a foundation of knowledge on heart disease, its diagnoses, its treatments and the ways to control and manage the disease.

Of course, your health is not just in your doctors' hands. It's in your own, and I can't help but return to the simple basics of prevention here. The key to a long, heart-healthy life and to model behaviour for your children and grandchildren is to reduce your risk in the future. Manage your diet, establish a routine of activity, quit smoking if you are a smoker, and control your diabetes and hypertension by making smart lifestyle choices and taking your medications. There's a very important, often life-saving, reason your doctor has given you prescriptions. Review your progress on the drugs and on your prevention plan. Discuss how well you're feeling in the bigger picture, not only with your cardiologist and family physician but also with your friends and loved ones. If you're constantly finding reasons to put off living a heart-healthier life, then "tomorrow" will never come. It's about prioritizing your health today and then maintaining your commitment throughout the ups and downs of life. Look ahead. The future is bright.

ACKNOWLEDGEMENTS

I'd like to thank several individuals for helping make this book possible. Kim Giles spent hundreds of hours typing and retyping and working with me on the manuscript. Her dedication, loyalty and organizational skills were an invaluable part of this process. She helped make this project a reality. Dr. Robert Chisholm provided thoughtful content advice as I embarked on the book. I am grateful for his support, guidance and friendship. Dr. Anthony Graham provided a scholarly review on behalf of the Heart and Stroke Foundation. Thank you, Tony, for your time and mentorship. Maryam Sanati worked with me tirelessly on many late-night editorial sessions. She helped keep my "voice" while making sense of complex medical concepts. Rick Broadhead provided essential advice on the process of writing a book. Kate Cassaday at HarperCollins approached me and asked me to write this book. Thank you, Kate, for your vision—I wouldn't have done it without you. Most importantly, all of my patients—your stories have shaped the case studies I have shared in this book. Even though a few personal details have been changed, your stories helped it come to life. Thank you all so much.

NOTES

Foreword

1 Statistics Canada, *Leading Causes of Death in Canada* (Ottawa: Statistics Canada, 2009).
2 Conference Board of Canada, *The Canadian Heart Health Strategy: Risk Factors and Future Cost Implications* (February 2010), www.conferenceboard.ca/e-library/abstract.aspx?did=3447.
3 Paula A. Johnson and JoAnn E. Manson, "How to Make Sure the Beat Goes On: Protecting a Woman's Heart," *Circulation* 111 (2005): e28–e33, doi: 10.1161/01.CIR.0000155364.54434.E6; World Health Organization, "Cardiovascular Diseases: Facts and Figures" (n.d.), www.euro.who.int/en/what-we-do/health-topics/noncommunicable-diseases/cardiovascular-diseases/facts-and-figures; and World Health Organization, Global Status Report on Noncommunicable Diseases 2010 (2011), www.who.int/nmh/publications/ncd_report2010/en.
4 Canadian Institute for Health Information, Hospital Morbidity Database, Hospitalization Data 2010: Most Reasonable Diagnosis.

Introduction

1 Statistics Canada, *Mortality, Summary List of Causes, 2008* (2011), catalogue no. 84F0209X, www.statcan.gc.ca/pub/84f0209x/84f0209x2008000-eng.pdf.
2 Conference Board of Canada, *The Canadian Heart Health Strategy: Risk Factors and Future Cost Implications* (February 2010), www.conferenceboard.ca/e-library/abstract.aspx?did=3447.

Chapter 2: Prediction and Risk Factors for Heart Disease

1 Salim Yusuf et al, "Global Burden of Cardiovascular Diseases—Part I: General Considerations, the Epidemiologic Transition, Risk Factors, and Impact of Urbanization," *Circulation* 104 (2001): 2746–2753.

2 Heart and Stroke Foundation, "Is 60 the New 70?" (Annual Report Card on Canadians' Health, 2006), http://www.heartandstroke.on.ca/site/c.pvI3IeNWJwE/b.3582055/k.F448/2006_Report_Card__Is_60_the_new_70.htm.

3 Statistics Canada, *Leading Causes of Death, Total Population, by Age Group and Sex, Canada* (2012), CANSIM database, Table 102–0561, www5.statcan.gc.ca/cansim/a26?lang=eng&retrLang=eng&id=1020561&paSer=&pattern=&stByVal=1&p1=1&p2=-1&tabMode=dataTable&csid.

4 Donald Lloyd-Jones et al, "Heart Disease and Stroke Statistics—2010 Update: A Report from the American Heart Association," *Circulation* 121 (2010): e46–e215.

5 Canadian Centre on Substance Abuse, *The Costs of Substance Abuse in Canada* (Ottawa: CCSA, 2002).

6 Donald Lloyd-Jones et al, "Heart Disease and Stroke Statistics—2010 Update: A Report from the American Heart Association," *Circulation* 121 (2010): e46–e215.

7 World Health Organization, "Tobacco," fact sheet no. 339 (May 2012), www.who.int/mediacentre/factsheets/fs339/en/index.html.

8 Judith MacKay, Michael Eriksen, and Omar Shafey, *The Tobacco Atlas* (Atlanta: American Cancer Society, 2006).

9 Health Canada, *Canadian Tobacco Use Monitoring Survey (CTUMS): Summary of Annual Results for 2010* (2011), www.hc-sc.gc.ca/hc-ps/tobac-tabac/research-recherche/stat/_ctums-esutc_2010/ann_summary-sommaire-eng.php.

10 Graham A. Colditz et al., "Cigarette Smoking and Risk of Stroke in Middle-Aged Women," *New England Journal of Medicine* 318, no. 15 (1988): 937–41.

11 Donald Lloyd-Jones et al, "Heart Disease and Stroke Statistics—2010 Update: A Report from the American Heart Association," *Circulation* 121 (2010): e46–e215.

12 American Heart Association, "What Your Cholesterol Levels Mean" (October 2012), www.heart.org/HEARTORG/Conditions/Cholesterol

/AboutCholesterol/What-Your-Cholesterol-Levels-Mean_UCM_305562_Article.jsp.

13 World Health Organization, *World Health Report 2002: Reducing Risks, Promoting Healthy Life* (2002), www.who.int/whr/2002/en/whr02_en.pdf: 58.

14 David R. MacLean, Andres Petrasovits and M. Nargundkhar, "Canadian Heart Health Surveys: A Profile of Cardiovascular Risk," *Canadian Medical Association Journal* 146 (1992): 1969–74.

15 Ramachandran S. Vasan et al., "Impact of High-Normal Blood Pressure on the Risk of Cardiovascular Disease," *New England Journal of Medicine* 345, no. 18 (2001): 1291–97.

16 American Heart Association, "Cardiovascular Disease & Diabetes" (February 2012), www.heart.org/HEARTORG/Conditions/Diabetes/WhyDiabetesMatters/Cardiovascular-Disease-Diabetes_UCM_313865_Article.jsp.

17 Peter Gaede et al., "Multifactorial Intervention and Cardiovascular Disease in Patients with Type 2 Diabetes," *New England Journal of Medicine* 348, no. 5 (2003): 383–93.

18 University of Oxford, "Moderate Obesity Takes Years Off Life Expectancy" (March 2009), www.ox.ac.uk/media/news_stories/2009/090317.html.

19 Steven D. Mittelman et al., "Adiposity Predicts Carotid Intima-Media Thickness in Healthy Children and Adolescents," *Journal of Pediatrics* 156, no. 4 (2010): 592–97.

20 M. Shields and M. S. Tremblay, "Sedentary Behavior and Obesity," *Health Reports* 19, no. 2 (2008): 19–30, quoted in Heart and Stroke Foundation, "Physical Activity, Heart Disease and Stroke," Position Statement (August 2011), www.heartandstroke.sk.ca/site/c.inKMILNlEmG/b.5265067/k.F8F8/Position_Statements_Physical_Activity_Heart_Disease_and_Stroke.htm.

21 P. M. Ridker et al, "Rosuvastatin to Prevent Vascular Events in Men and Women with Elevated C-Reactive Protein," *New England Journal of Medicine* 359, no. 21 (2008): 2195–207.

22 W. B. Kannel and D. L. McGee, "Diabetes and Cardiovascular Disease: The Framingham Study," *Journal of the American Medical Association* 241 (1979): 2035–38.

23 National Heart, Lung and Blood Institute and Boston University, "Framington Heart Study: Risk Score Profiles," www.framinghamheartstudy.org/risk/index.html.

Chapter 3: Women and Heart Disease

1 Heart and Stroke Foundation, "Time to Bridge the Gender Gap" (Annual Report Card on Canadians' Health, 2007), http://www.heartandstroke.com/site/apps/nlnet/content2.aspx?c=ikIQLcMWJtE&b=4955951&ct=4512811.

2 A. S. Bierman et al, "Cardiovascular Diseases," *Project for an Ontario Women's Health Evidence-Based Report* 1, A. S. Bierman, ed. (Toronto, 2009), powerstudy.ca.

3 JoAnn E. Manson et al. for the Women's Health Initiative Investigators, "Estrogen Plus Progestin and the Risk of Coronary Heart Disease," *New England Journal of Medicine* 349, no. 6 (2003): 523–34.

4 Deborah Grady et al, HERS Research Group, "Cardiovascular Disease Outcomes During 6.8 Years of Hormone Therapy: Heart and Estrogen/Progestin Replacement Study Follow-Up (HERS II)," *Journal of the American Medical Association* 288, no. 1 (Jul 2002): 49–57.

5 N. K, Wenger and J. Stamler, "The Coronary Drug Project: Implications for Clinical Care," *Primary Care* 4, no. 2 (June 1977): 247–53.

Chapter 4: Primary Prevention

1 S. Yusuf et al, "Effect of Potentially Modifiable Risk Factors Associated with Myocardial Infarction in 52 Countries (the INTERHEART study): Case-Control Study," *Lancet* 364 (2004): 937–52.

2 Majid Ezzati et al., "Role of Smoking in Global and Regional Cardiovascular Mortality," *Circulation* 112 (2005): 489–97.

3 Nancy A. Rigotti et al., "Bupropion for Smokers Hospitalized with Acute Cardiovascular Disease," *American Journal of Medicine* 119, no. 12 (2006): 1080–87.

4 Nancy A. Rigotti et al., "Efficacy and Safety of Varenicline for Smoking Cessation in Patients with Cardiovascular Disease: A Randomized Trial," *Circulation* 121, no. 2 (2010): 221–29.

5 S. J. Nielsen and B.M. Popkin, "Changes in Beverage Intake Between 1977 and 2001," *American Journal of Preventive Medicine* 27, no. 3 (2004): 205–10.

6 Kuklina, Elena V., Paula W. Yoon and Nora L. Keenan, "Prevalence of Coronary Heart Disease Risk Factors and Screening for High Cholesterol Levels Among Young Adults, United States, 1999–2006," *Annals of Family Medicine* 8 (2010): 327–33.

7 Canadian Society for Exercise Physiology, "Canadian Physical Activity Guidelines," www.csep.ca/english/view.asp?x=804.

8 Frank M. Sacks et al., "Comparison of Weight-Loss Diets with Different Compositions of Fat, Protein, and Carbohydrates," *New England Journal of Medicine* 360, no. 9 (2009): 859–73.

9 National Heart Lung and Blood Institute: Health Information Network, "5 Steps to a Healthy Weight," *Health-e Actions* (October 15, 2010), http://hp2010.nhlbihin.net/joinhin/news/consumer/ConsumerWtLossReality.htm.

10 Bret H. Goodpaster et al., "Effects of Diet and Physical Activity Interventions on Weight Loss and Cardiometabolic Risk Factors in Severely Obese Adults: A Randomized Trial," *Journal of the American Medical Association* 304, no. 16 (2010): 1795–802.

11 National Heart Lung and Blood Institute, "What Is the DASH Eating Plan?" (July 2012), www.nhlbi.nih.gov/health/health-topics/topics/dash.

12 N. R. Campbell et al, "Canadian Hypertension Education Program: The Science Supporting New 2011 CHEP Recommendations with an Emphasis on Health Advocacy and Knowledge Translation," *Canadian Journal of Cardiology* 27, no. 4 (2011): 407–14.

13 Nigel S. Beckett et al.; HYVET Study Group, "Treatment of Hypertension in Patients 80 Years of Age or Older," *New England Journal of Medicine* 358, no. 18 (2008): 1887–98.

Chapter 5: Symptoms

1 John G. Canto et al., NRMI Investigators, "Association of Age and Sex with Myocardial Infarction Symptom Presentation and In-Hospital Mortality," *Journal of the American Medical Association* 307, no. 8 (2012): 813–22.

Chapter 7: Other Important Tests for the Heart

1 Tanja Meyer et al., "Radiation Exposure and Dose Reduction Measures in Cardiac CT," *Current Cardiovascular Imaging Reports* 1, no. 2 (2008): 133–40, doi:10.1007/s12410-008-0020-3.

2 C. M. Ballantyne et al, "Effect of Rosuvastatin Therapy on Coronary Artery Stenoses Assessed by Quantitative Coronary Angiography: A Study to Evaluate the Effect of Rosuvastatin on Intravascular Ultrasound-Derived Coronary Atheroma Burden," *Circulation* 117, no. 19 (2008): 2458–66.

Chapter 8: What Your Diagnosis Means: Coronary Heart Disease

1 Beth L. Abramson et al; Canadian Cardiovascular Society, "Canadian Cardiovascular Society Consensus Conference: Peripheral Arterial Disease—Executive Summary," *Canadian Journal of Cardiology* 21, no. 12 (2005): 997–1006.

Chapter 9: What Your Diagnosis Means: Non-Coronary Heart Disease

1 Alan S. Go et al., "Prevalence of Diagnosed Atrial Fibrillation in Adults: National Implications for Rhythm Management and Stroke Prevention—the AnTicoagulation and Risk Factors in Atrial Fibrillation (ATRIA) Study," *Journal of the American Medical Association* 285, no. 18 (2001): 2370–75.

2 Robert A. Fowler et al., "Sex-and Age-Based Differences in the Delivery and Outcomes of Critical Care," Canadian Medical Association Journal 177, no. 12 (2007): 1513–19.

Chapter 10: Treatments for Coronary Heart Disease

1 A. S. Bierman et al, "Cardiovascular Diseases," *Project for an Ontario Women's Health Evidence-Based Report* 1, A. S. Bierman, ed. (Toronto, 2009) powerstudy.ca.

2 P. M. Ridker et al, "Cardiovascular Benefits and Diabetes Risks of Statin Therapy in Primary Prevention: An Analysis from the JUPITER Trial," *Lancet* 380, no. 9841 (2012): 565–71.

3 David Hasdai et al., "Effect of Smoking Status on the Long-Term Outcome After Successful Percutaneous Coronary Revascularization," *New England Journal of Medicine* 336, no. 11 (1997): 755–61.

4 Beth L. Abramson and Nancy Reballato, "Smoking Cessation," *Cardiology Rounds* 10, no. 9 (2005), www.cardiologyrounds.ca.

5 Jeffrey L. Anderson et al., "ACC/AHA 2007 Guidelines for the Management of Patients with Unstable Angina/Non-ST-Elevation Myocardial Infarction: A Report of the American College of Cardiology/American Heart Association Task Force on Practice Guidelines," *Circulation* 116 (2007): e148–e304.

6 W. E. Boden et al; COURAGE Trial Research Group, "Optimal Medical Therapy with or without PCI for Stable Coronary Disease," *New England Journal of Medicine* 356, no. 15 (2007); 1503–16.

7 Heart and Stroke Foundation, The 2010 Guidelines for CPR and Emergency Cardiovascular Care (2010), www.heartandstroke.ca/CPRguidelines.

Chapter 11: Treatments for Arrhythmias

1 David J. Gladstone et al., "Potentially Preventable Strokes in High-Risk Patients with Atrial Fibrillation Who Are Not Adequately Anticoagulated," *Stroke* 40, no. 1 (2009): 235–40.

Chapter 12: Treatment of Heart Failure

1 R. S. Bhatia et al, "Outcome of Heart Failure with Preserved Ejection Fraction in a Population-Based Study," New England Journal of Medicine 355, no. 3 (2006): 260–69.

2 Douglas S. Lee et al., "Improved Outcomes with Early Collaborative Care of Ambulatory Heart Failure Patients Discharged from the Emergency Department," *Circulation* 122, no. 18 (2010): 1806–14.

3 A. S. Bierman et al, "Cardiovascular Diseases," *Project for an Ontario Women's Health Evidence-Based Report* 1, A. S. Bierman, ed. (Toronto, 2009), powerstudy.ca.

Chapter 14: Secondary Prevention and Cardiac Rehab

1 Rod S. Taylor et al., "Exercise-Based Rehabilitation for Patients with Coronary Heart Disease: Systematic Review and Meta-Analysis of Randomized Controlled Trials," *American Journal of Medicine* 116 (2004): 682–92.

2 Heart and Stroke Foundation, *Recovery Road*, www.heartandstroke.com/site/c.ikIQLcMWJtE/b.3751099/k.C320/Heart_disease__Recovery_Road.htm.

3 Chris Simpson et al., "Consensus Conference 2003: Assessment of the Cardiac Patient for Fitness to Drive and Fly—Executive Summary," *Canadian Journal of Cardiology* 20, no. 13 (2004): 1313–23.

4 The Heart Outcomes Prevention Evaluation Study Investigators, "Effects of an Angiotensin-Converting–Enzyme Inhibitor, Ramipril, on Cardiovascular Events in High-Risk Patients," *New England Journal of Medicine* 342 (2000): 145–53.

Chapter 16: Innovations

1 Martin B. Leon et al.; PARTNER Trial Investigators, "Transcatheter Aortic-Valve Implantation for Aortic Stenosis in Patients Who Cannot Undergo Surgery," *New England Journal of Medicine* 363, no. 17 (2010): 1597–607.

2 Elizabeth G. Nabel, "Gene Therapy for Cardiovascular Disease," *Circulation* 91 (1995): 541–48.

3 Human Genome Project Information, Pharmacogenomics (July 2012), http://www.ornl.gov/sci/techresources/Human_Genome/home.shtml.

INDEX

B

D

G

H

I

J

K

L

M

N

O

P

Q

R

T

U

V

W

X

Y

Z